AWAKENING

AWAKENING

FROM THE SEXUALLY ADDICTED MIND:

A GUIDE TO COMPASSIONATE RECOVERY

DARRIN FORD

LMFT, CSAT-S, MBATT-S

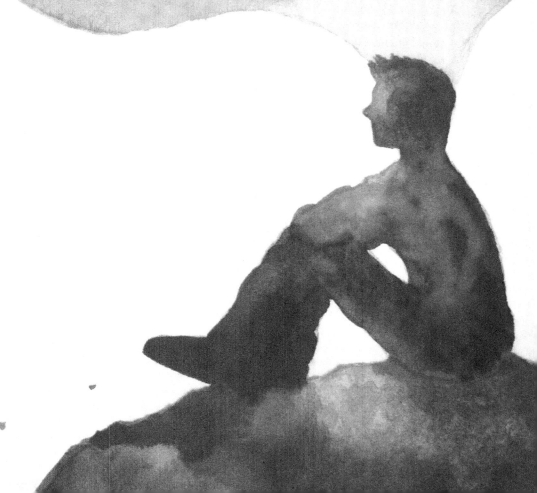

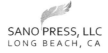

SANO PRESS, LLC
LONG BEACH, CA

Copyright © 2019 by Darrin Ford LMFT, CSAT-S, MBATT-S
All rights reserved. No part of this publication may be used or reproduced, stored or entered into a retrieval system, transmitted, photocopied, recorded, or otherwise reproduced in any form by any mechanical or electronic means, without the prior written permission of the authors and Sano Press, with the exception of brief quotations for the purposes of review articles.

1st Edition

Front cover image © BenStudioPRO #233311369. Book design & layout by Chris Bordey. Editing by Christian Quebral & Chris Bordey. Sano feather ™ Sano Press LLC.

PRINT ISBN-13: 978-1-7339222-2-7
EPUB ISBN-13: 978-1-7339222-5-8

Dedication

I dedicate this book to the village of powerful, independent women in my life:

- My mother, Barbara, who has always taught me to work hard, be consistent, and live honorably.
- My stepmother, Laura, who would tell me, "You have the gift of gab!"
- My sister, Debbie, who taught me to be tenacious and focused.
- My Aunt Joanne—for her support and encouragement in telling me, "That's okay, you will get it!"
- My former therapist, Sharon Neisell, who taught me that not only is it okay to cry, but that crying is a sign of emotional health.
- My business partner, colleague, and friend Mari A. Lee, "The Counselor's Coach," who has held me to task and organized the chaos of my mind.

Without my tribe, I would not be who I am today.

CONTENTS

INTRODUCTION 08

CH. 1 MIND 11

CH. 2 ACCEPTANCE 26

CH. 3 MEDITATION 38

CH. 4 METTA 77

CH. 5 AWARENESS 94

CH. 6 HONESTY 127

CH. 7 SEX 145

CH. 8 EQUANIMITY 166

REFERENCES 178

ABOUT THE AUTHOR 185

INTRODUCTION

Two main factors led me to write this book. The first is the all too common story of culture teaching us to suppress, obliterate, or distract ourselves from the experience of human emotion. This fundamental misunderstanding that we need to distance ourselves from painful emotions has paved the way for continuous suffering on a global scale, propagating trauma and addiction. Imagine if a global community could sit in the distress of an emotion long enough to allow for awareness, understanding, and acceptance to arise from their emotional experience.

The second driving factor for writing this book is to educate people in the field of recovery treatment about the brain, which is not only *cause*; it is also *effect*. When we choose to focus our mind on building healthy habits for dealing with emotional pain, we construct (or reinforce) neurological pathways, which brings about healing. The pathways we don't use—like the ones we created or enhanced with addiction—diminish. When we move focus away from old behaviors, the body begins to deconstruct them—though they are never fully gone.

The manifestation of "mental health disorders," like addiction, is often not a disorder at all, but a natural outcome to the causes and conditions of one's life—a reaction to dealing with unprocessed pain. For those who believe they are fundamentally broken because they are addicts, it is my hope that reading this book will allow you to have a compassionate awareness that you are not, nor have you ever been "broken." You are having a normal reaction to traumatic events in your life. Though biology plays a role, it is my experience that we can overcome our genetic predisposition to a considerable extent through mindful practice, disciplined habits, and a relentless application of compassion. There has been (and always will be) recovery available to you.

You must begin to see that the addict mind was trying to care for you, but this attempt at self-love was destructive, to say the least. This book is a guide to helping you learn to love yourself and those around you in a healthy manner. To do this, you must gain intimacy with yourself by building tolerance to the experience of your emotions. There is no shortcut here. There is only a long path that leads to a place of love—a belonging you never thought possible.

With compassion and respect,
—Darrin

Chapter 1

MIND

On the right side of the room, we set up our pine tree, adorned with red bows, wrapped with golden garland, twinkling lights, and rows of popcorn. We worked hard on our Christmas tree, and it turned out so pretty that it filled me with joy.

To the left, I saw two silhouetted figures, backlit by a wall of windows. I could not hear what they were saying but could see mouths moving and fingers pointing. A phone receiver appeared in one of the hands and was smashed into the head of the other figure. The hand rose again and struck once more. As one shadow fell to the ground, the other walked away. That's when I saw the silhouette was wearing a green sweater that belonged to my father. He was holding the phone receiver while my mother collapsed on our mid-seventies, brown shag carpet in a pool of blood in front of our beautiful Christmas tree—red bows and all.

This is my first memory of childhood. Not long after this event, around the time I was four years old, my mother divorced my father. My sister and I stayed with my mother, and we would visit my father on select weekends.

When I was eleven years old, I decided I wanted to move in with my father. I had my reasons, some of which were unconscious at the time. I called from a payphone inside of a train station-themed McDonald's in Barstow, California, where my parents would meet to exchange us kids on the weekends. My stepmother, Laura, stood by my side as I made the call. I felt scared to tell my mother. I remember the horror in her voice. I can only imagine the fear she felt hearing it.

The law allowed me to move in with my father, so my mother had no choice but to let me. I lived with my father and stepmother for the next three eye-opening years.

The last day I lived with my biological father was, again, at Christmas time. We were setting up that wonderful tree, and it wasn't balancing correctly. My stepmother and father went into the garage to argue. My stepbrother, Jeff, who was two years my senior and I were in the kitchen listening. Jeff opened the door between the kitchen and the garage, and to our horror, we witnessed my father spit in Laura's face and punch her. Blood flew across the white bow of my father's speedboat.

My father noticed us and was stunned that we had witnessed the whole thing. He ordered Jeff to close the door. As

CHAPTER 1: MIND

he did, my stepmother Laura ran to the car in the driveway. She pulled at the door handles of her white Grand Prix with the red velvet interior, but the door was locked. I saw her car keys on the kitchen counter. I was filled with a desire to grab them and run them to her, but my father was between us—I would have had to make it through him somehow.

I assessed the situation, and my mind told me that it was hopeless. I turned around and walked up the stairs, back to my room as if nothing had happened. In reality, I was shocked and horrified. For decades after this event, I carried such shame—the word coward repeatedly arose in my mind.

Traumatic events programmed my mind as I was growing up. Not only did I witness my father abuse my mother and stepmother, but I was also raped twice and molested throughout my childhood. With these experiences, I developed a particular lens through which I saw the world.

My programming taught me that distressing emotions were negative. Any emotion other than love, joy, and passion were bad. In order to avoid distress, I repressed, suppressed, and cut myself off from shame, guilt, pain, anger, and fear.

I acted out dramatically using drugs, sex, and money to keep the "bad" emotions at bay, causing a feedback loop where the harder I tried to avoid the rising tide of negative emotions, the less I could feel the positive ones. Emotions create thoughts, thoughts coalesce into beliefs, beliefs manifest into behaviors, behaviors are practiced into habits, and habits become our destiny. The mind—erroneously thinking this is what we need to survive—supports these habits, no matter how self-destructive they are. While in our addiction, the chasm between emotions and oneself only widens. Our attempts to numb our emotions intensify and our behaviors become increasingly extreme.

As I grew older, the chasm between these emotions and myself became so wide that the other emotions—love, joy, and passion—could also no longer be felt. When we numb ourselves to one emotion, we eventually numb ourselves to all emotions. This pattern is not unique in the human experience. We all do this to some extent when we are confronted with traumatic, emotional experiences. Ironically, the more we avoid an emotion, the more powerful it becomes.

This avoidance is based on the environmental programming we receive growing up, though genetics does play a part. As a result of my programming, I could not trust what my mind told me. My upbringing taught me not to trust anything or anyone, including myself. If someone said they loved me, I believed they were going to hurt me.

To heal, I needed to go against my judgment and ask for help. I had to go against my beliefs if I ever wanted to recover and allow myself to feel anything again. This is where you are, and this is where recovery begins.

Recovery is a lifelong practice of reprogramming your mind, of creating a new lens through which to see the world. You will need to relate to your shame, guilt, pain, anger, fear, joy, passion, and love in a way you have never done before. You must look at the various beliefs you have about these emotions. If you are going to know yourself, you must know your mind—the tool we use to interact with the world.

Mind

"I was not in my right mind" is a phrase commonly used to explain uncharacteristic behaviors, but what exactly is mind? It depends on who you ask. There are many definitions and schools of thought. The one we will examine in this book is based on Buddhist psychology. According to the New College of the University of Toronto website:

> Buddhist psychology is primarily about self-knowledge, finding out more about who you are, understanding your decisions, actions, thoughts, feelings, etc. It is an expression of the Delphic dictum *Know Thyself* and the injunction that transformative spiritual paths throughout time and geography have demanded as the central ingredient in authentic happiness.

Buddhist psychology is 'radical,' as it aims to challenge your worldview (as all authentic spirituality and psychology does). It is radical in that it addresses the basis or foundation of our psychological functioning, our sense of who we are, and our relationships with others and with the world. As a result, the fruit of applying the psychological insights of the Buddha requires diligence, perseverance and discernment as they will naturally encounter the resistances and obstacles inherent in our conditioned nature.

Think of the mind as a sensory organ. Just as you have eyes for seeing blue, a nose for smelling rain, a tongue for tasting water, and skin for feeling warmth—you also have a mind for compiling information. Your mind takes in data from your environment and formulates hypotheses based on past data (your memories), and the information presented to the brain at the time of perception.

We always say things like "I am angry," or "I think you are wrong," but who is this "I"? The *I* is not the thinking—if you were the thinking, then how could you have the awareness that you were, in fact, thinking whatever it was you were thinking?

If the mind is a sense organ that produces thought, and you are not thoughts, then you cannot be mind. Yet we make the mistake of claiming our thoughts as our identities.

To put it another way, if you looked across the room and saw a waterfall, would you say, "I am waterfall?" Of course, not. This sounds ridiculous. The same goes for the mind. The mind is heavily influenced by the data it has been programmed with. You can think of your mind much like the operating system of a computer. The computer itself is not the operating system, as you are not your mind.

You are the awareness that observes the mind. This is important to understand when it comes to addiction. If you can detach yourself from the idea that you are your emotions and thoughts, then when you have a craving, you can let it rise, crest, and fall into oblivion. You can learn to watch your thoughts without reacting to them. We will delve more deeply into this later. For now, let's examine the mechanics of the mind. The following are the stages the mind goes through to create beliefs, and thus actions:

1. Mind senses data.

2. Mind cross-checks data with memory.

3. Mind creates an emotion (If the emotion is perceived as aversive, the body/mind responds aversely).

4. Mind begins to assess the emotion and forms thoughts or ideas.

5. Mind collapses thoughts/ideas into belief.

6. Mind molds belief into a hypothesis.

7. Behavior has the potential to manifest.

8. Behaviors are practiced into habits (Addiction).

9. Habits become our destiny.

Beliefs, and thus actions, are associated with the limbic system, the impulse center and the cortex of the brain. (I use the idea of the impulse center of the brain loosely; a neuroscientist would gasp and shake his head, but for the sake of discussion, it will suffice.) The idea that the brain determines the mind is controversial in scientific circles. However, an argument can be made that the focus on rewards (even harmful rewards) can trigger neuroplasticity—the brain's ability to reorganize itself in response to events.

In fact, there is evidence of this all around us. At this very moment, you are focusing consciousness and awareness on the words of this page. The ideas presented here are generating connections among neurons; a memory is being created, and you are learning. This is done when you focus the mind on organizing and coordinating the data you receive.

The Three Poisons

With addiction, we have a mind that has misunderstood—or is in delusion—about the positive effect of the behavior or substance we are addicted to. To heal, we must understand certain states of mind that are directly correlated with suffering. In Buddhist psychology, these mindstates are called the three poisons. (When I bring up the idea of Buddhist psychology, I am looking at it first as a scientist, then as a Buddhist. I am basing my definition off of empirical evidence, not belief.) Three specific states of mind are important for us to know about in recovery.

1. *Mindstate of attachment.* The craving mind, to use the 12-step adage, "Wants what it wants, when it wants it." It infinitely desires what it believes is gratifying, and it is never satisfied for long. The mind can also attach to other people, claiming it cannot be without them. The mind will say it wants more, but the end is always the same—suffering, pain, and loss of control over one's life.

2. *Mindstate of avoidance or aversion.* This state of mind is associated with willfully not wanting to deal with the reality of what is. It is a defense mechanism we have used throughout the years to avoid things that the mind believes is somehow not good. The natural and normal human response of pushing away emotional pain is an example of the aversive mind at work. Another example is how we sometimes tell ourselves not to cry or to suck it up. This can stem from parents instilling this mentality in their children, by saying things such as, "Stop crying, or I will give you something to cry about." In this case, the parent is utilizing an aversive mindset to push away their own

discomfort with a certain emotional state by telling the child to stop feeling whatever the child is feeling.

When I was in my mid-thirties, I lost my father. It took a very long time to accept the reality that he was gone. For over a year and a half, his number remained on my phone. This is another example of the aversive mind at work. As human beings, we push away the pain of loss. With addiction, our mind will tell us, "You cannot handle this pain, so you have to use at least a little/act out just this one last time." The outcome of the addictive cycle is always the same; we end up in despair, and our lives become unmanageable. This can happen so quickly within the mind that we may be ignorant of it.

3. *Mindstate of ignorance.* Here, the mind simply does not know. For example, at age thirteen, you don't understand that drinking alcohol is harmful or addictive. If you are around family members who are struggling with addiction and are always drinking, your focus may be on drinking. You will do everything to get all the alcohol you can. Another example: if you are sexualized at a young age, you will not understand the negative consequences related to sex. This is why we have laws to protect children. Thus, your mind will tell you that you want more sex because it believes it's the best thing since sliced bread, and of course, sexual

contact is euphoric in nature. As a result, addiction develops a foothold. I cannot tell you how many people come into my office who are victims of sexual abuse, and they (especially men) say, "But I wanted it." I explain to them two things:

- A biological reaction (e.g. an erection) does not mean you understand sex at that age.

- Even if you, as a child, actively looked for sex, it is up to the adults around you to explain and educate you about engaging in the behavior in a safe and healthy way. Your brain was not fully developed yet. In fact, our prefrontal cortex does not fully develop until about the age of twenty-five. There is no way you can be fully aware of the impact of the choices you are making. Thus, you are in a mind of ignorance.

IGNORANCE, DELUSION, DENIAL

Before continuing, we should describe the differences between the following terms.

- *Ignorance* is simply not knowing.

- *Delusion* is knowing but misunderstanding.

- *Denial* is knowing and understanding, but not accepting.

With addiction, these mindstates play an important role since they allow the mind to stay trapped in an endless, unmanageable cycle that will not cease until the emotional pain can no longer be ignored or until a person dies. Just as people die from alcoholism or drug overdoses, people die every year from sex addiction through choking, suffocation, sexually transmitted diseases, or auto accidents (to name a few).

The mind is the single most powerful tool we have to gain information in our lives. Addiction has corrupted the operating system of the addict, and we must work to take it back.

Neuroplasticity

Neuroplasticity is the process of focusing consciously to generate new neural pathways. When we focus on constructing new, healthy neural connections, we are simultaneously removing our focus from harmful ones. The breakdown of unused neural circuits ensues, and this is all made possible with the use of our attention. When it comes to the human body, the phrase "use it or lose it" is true, and it is the basis of learning. What we choose to use will stay, and what we don't use will wither. However, it's not as black and white as it sounds, and addiction further complicates the process. The neurological pathways of impulsivity are strengthened in an addict. The human body believes that these strengthened neural connections are vital to existence and devotes more energy to these pathways. As a result, the addict's body believes that the avoidance of distressing emotions through the activation of impulsive behaviors is important for the organism's survival.

When a child is born, the most developed part of their limbic system is referred to as the reptilian brain. In the evolution of the human brain, the reptilian brain is the oldest part and represents the youngest part of our concept of self. A child being held by its mother or father is not aware that they are a separate entity from the parent; they simply absorb the ambient emotionality in the room like a sponge in water. Let's say a child lives in a highly stressful environment, and an emotion such as fear is prevalent. The pathways related to fear in the child will be strengthened, and as the child grows older, fear will play a bigger role in their life, and they become highly reactionary to their environment.

The prefrontal cortex is involved in logic, reasoning, and understanding the consequences of one's choices. It allows us to pause and sit with stressful emotions prior to taking action. When a child grows up in an environment dominated by fear, the prolonged stress inhibits the growth of the prefrontal cortex, resulting in a child (or even an adult) who does not see the consequences of their choices. Simultaneously, because the prefrontal cortex has not fully developed, the child will be incapable of sitting with their uncomfortable emotions. They will act out in ways to numb their feelings. As their effort to not feel progresses into adulthood, vast parts of their lives are neglected, chaos ensues, and addiction flourishes.

The good news is that studies prove the addicted mind can be rewired. Concentrated effort, (like meditation) has been shown to affect the amygdala—the part of the brain dedicated to aggressiveness and impulsivity. This effort weakens neural connections in that area while simultaneously strengthening neural connections in the prefrontal cortex. This was measured with an fMRI study in which they captured images of the size and neural density of participants' brains before an 8-week mindfulness-based stress reduction course and again after the intervention. The concept of rewiring the mind is further illustrated by studies on adults who struggle with ADHD. After the same 8-week mindfulness-based stress reduction course, all of the participants displayed a marked improvement in behavior functions. This is neural plasticity at work.

At *Mindful Centers for Addiction and Trauma Therapy*, we actively use mindfulness-based techniques to assist clients in changing their addictive behaviors with significant success. There is no limit to our ability to harness the power of neuroplasticity. I recently watched a video of an adolescent boy who took two minutes and thirty seconds to look at a Rubik's Cube from all different angles. Shortly after, he was blindfolded, and in less than two minutes, he solved the cube without looking at it. The only way he was able to do this was with practice. What you place your attention on will be prioritized in the brain and mind. As a result, the brain devotes energy to what you pay attention to, and the amount of attention spent is a determining factor in the strength of that neural circuit.

Of course, there are limits—not all of us can solve a Rubik's Cube in under two minutes while blindfolded. But if we are struggling with compulsive behaviors, we can utilize our attention and practice tools that will help us live differently. With addiction, we used attention and focus to solidify certain behaviors, and this now needs to shift. The many feats an addict overcomes to serve their addiction is proof that they can live a life in recovery. This is accomplished by generating new, healthy neural connections while diminishing established, destructive neural pathways.

It is important to note that these addictive neural pathways can never be completely removed. Addicts will have to participate in a supportive community for lifelong recovery—a daunting sounding feat—but one that is completely attainable if we choose to use our minds for it.

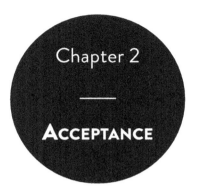

Chapter 2

ACCEPTANCE

I had just spread the towel over the white pavement in front of my house. With my cordless phone in hand, I laid back to bask in the July afternoon sun, sizzling my skin to a golden brown. At sixteen-years-old, friends and appearance were top priorities.

As I got comfortable, a police car turned into our forked driveway. Veering to the left would bring you to my grandmother's home while veering to the right would send you to my parents'. We lived on the outskirts of town where very few cars drove by, much less police cars. I was perplexed and curious.

I sat up as the officer got out of the car. He approached me and asked if my parents were home. I told him they weren't and asked if there was something I could help him with. He shook his head, thanked me, got back into his car, and left. Having the short attention span of a teenager, the cop quickly left my mind.

A few days later, I came home from school and found my mother and father with the same officer, sitting at the dining room table. I set my books on the counter, feeling the thick air of distress in the room. When my mom asked me to come to the table, I felt tingles run up my back, through my stomach and into my throat. My stomach was in knots, and my shoulders tensed. In a timid voice, I asked, "What's wrong?" Every last pore on my body oozed fear and terror, and I had no hope of managing this level of emotion, as no child would.

Officer Rodriguez addressed me. He told me that the police had some recordings of disturbing phone calls, and those calls had been traced to my bedroom phone line. At that moment, I knew what this was about: I had been making sexually obscene (and what I thought were anonymous) phone calls to a classmate.

The officer continued, "We would not want to cause your family embarrassment, and those who have received the calls have agreed not to press charges. That being said, this must stop."

Officer Rodriguez was a family friend. My family was well-connected where we lived. In small towns, everyone knows each other, and if you had a stepfather (such as I did) who graduated from high school and lived his whole life in that town, you were one of the *insiders*—we received special treatment. At insider parties, where underage drinking occurred, cops who disrupted the festivities would simply tell us to go home. Outsiders, on the other hand, were busted and escorted to the local police station. For insiders, this created a mindset of invulnerability, which was abruptly ending for me at this moment.

My mother turned to me and asked, "Darrin, why?"

I said nothing before I broke down in tears. The deeply wounded boy buried inside of me—the damaged child who was repeatedly molested and the teenager who was raped—was now being seen by others. I answered in the most honest and truthful way I could. "I don't know! I don't know!" I covered my face with my hands as I sobbed. My mother held me. I had no idea what my father was thinking, and to this day, I still don't know.

I went to my room, and my parents continued talking with Officer Rodriguez for awhile. When he left, my mother came to me and asked how I was doing.

I answered, "Okay, I guess."

"We talked to the officer, and you are not going to get in any trouble over this. But you can never do this again. I have no idea what you said on the phone, but I know it was bad enough for the police to not let me hear the tapes."

The victim of my sexually obscene phone calls was a school friend. Officer Rodriguez told my friend not to tell anyone, and I had not considered the possibility he would. But when I went to school the next day, everyone was talking about it. My best friend came into class, sat next to me, and said, "Dude, you should hear what they are saying about you out there."

I replied, "What are you talking about?"

At that moment, my mind split. I buried the inner child and wounded teenager, who had briefly appeared in the room with Officer Rodriguez, so far down that he would not show himself again for years. When he did emerge, I had no idea who he was, what he was, or why he existed, and my addiction flourished.

If I had the ability back then to accept that wounded child, and had I been able to sit with the shame and fear, which were ingrained into my soul, I would have saved myself decades of emotional turmoil and catastrophe. But I was not capable, and no kids of that age are.

I'm still getting familiar with that wounded child to this day. Except now, I accept him—for better or worse—and we are a pair, marching through this thing called life. We will never be able to separate, so all we can do is love each other.

What is acceptance?

The moment that we seek help for our addiction is the beginning of acceptance, where we meet the inner part of our soul that we buried to not feel painful emotions. We welcome the guilt, pain, shame, and fear that we have denied. Acceptance of who we are—the flawed, pained, perfectly imperfect people we are—is essential for healing. Does acceptance mean we will not have consequences? Absolutely not. We must all pay the interest on the addiction credit card we have been charging up, and that starts with self-acceptance.

If we are to align with honesty and cultivate recovery, we must accept the totality of the damage we have done to those we love and to ourselves. We can no longer put up rationalizations. We have to acknowledge that others are in distress as a result of our behaviors.

The process of acceptance is not about feeling better. It is about getting better. To do so, we must unequivocally (without pretense and image control), accept the same pain, guilt, and fear that we have caused. If we have participated in addictive behaviors, we must accept that fact. We must own that we are capable of this. We must choose to love that part of ourselves and find a way to cultivate compassion. If we do not, we will be lost forever.

In the process of self-acceptance, there is no room for self-judgment. You are not good or bad for what you have done, you are not more or less valuable, and you are not more or less lovable. All of these dualities are nonsense. You are lovable, not for what you have or haven't done, you are lovable for who you are. Opening to the shame, pain, fear, and guilt in one's life is not about judgments—it's about feelings.

Feelings are not thoughts as much as they are energetic states that arise out of the body and the lizard brain. Emotions are the voice of the inner child. We have to attune and be present with them. No emotion is good or bad. All emotions are natural states—they arise out of the reality that as humans, we feel.

We have been indoctrinated with harmful ideas about feelings. Our culture has informed us that:

- We are bad for feeling.
- It is wrong to feel.

These are lies that have cost you, me, and society dearly. If we are to accept ourselves, we must accept the emotions that we feel. The fantasy of the strong, unfeeling cowboy must end.

This idea of radical acceptance is not an event—it is a process practiced over a lifetime. It is done only through compassionate approaches to the emotional energy that arises. We must first:

- See the emotion.
- Identify it.
- Be present with it.

- Recognize its transient nature.

We must be aware that various situations in our lives elicit emotions without warning. If we are mindful, we can recognize this fact, sit with the emotion, let it dissipate, and react to the situation constructively. Failing to do this, we become impulsive, reactionary—and later on—haunted with discomfort, which is pronounced with the regret of our behavior.

The Most Difficult Part of Recovery

The fact that we are people who feel, who have been wounded, who are lovable but struggle with addiction is hard to accept. We are people who have hurt others, helped others, hurt ourselves, helped ourselves—and we will always be lovable. You are lovable!

I can tell you repeatedly that you are lovable. You can tell yourself you are lovable. Those around you can tell you the same. But it may mean nothing to you. Until you accept it as fact, it will continue to mean nothing. When I say accept it, I do not mean have a rational perspective of it. To have acceptance of your lovability, you must know—not believe—that you are lovable.

Knowing or Believing

The difference between knowing and believing is a difficult concept for many people to grasp. Psychiatrist Carl Jung was once asked in an interview if he believed "something" to be true. His response left me perplexed, and my confusion lasted quite a long time. He replied, "Either I know a thing, and then I know it—I don't need to believe it."

When we *believe* something, there is still the possibility of it not being true. We hold an "opinion" about it. However, to *know* something is to hold it as truth. Not to hope it is true, but to hold it as true. When we look up at the blue sky, we know it is the sun that lights the Earth. This is an example of a fact, and therefore, not a belief.

The same is true for the concept of loving one's self. We are not truly aligned with reality until we are able to have the same certainty about our lovability. Moving into this space requires practice. Take time each day to focus on the idea of love. Behave compassionately towards others, including yourself.

I always tell my clients at the end of each therapy session, "Be gentle with yourself. After all, throughout your life in active addiction, were you not extremely harsh to yourself?" Your mind was filled with unbridled judgment toward yourself and others. You have always been angry. Angry at someone or something for not having or being what you want. You have always been upset with yourself for multiple reasons. Your internal dialogue was critical. This mindset spins your wheels into the same chaotic mess of addiction you had always been in. It is time to stop and cultivate gentle, but firm, loving, kindness.

This cannot be done if you allow the addictive mind to dictate your actions. Instead, you must set clear boundaries for yourself and accept the limits of your humanity. You must take care of yourself by setting a clear schedule around when you wake, eat, sleep, rest, and love—all parts of practicing recovery. For instance, you cannot work 80 hours a week. You need to treat yourself in a loving manner by getting quality, adequate sleep each night, eating nutritionally-balanced meals, brushing and flossing your teeth after eating, and making sure your home is a safe and peaceful place to come home to.

THE GIFT OF ACCEPTANCE

As stated before, acceptance is not a single event; it is a process. The mind tells us that if we choose to accept an event, then we must be able to move on. However, true acceptance is to recognize that you have experienced a betrayal or violation, and that you will have strong feelings and emotions as a result.

I hold powerful emotions of anger toward the man that raped me. My mind envisions bodily injury befalling him by my hands. If I was to say to myself that it was bad or wrong to have these thoughts, I would go down a path of self-denial, which would result in a non-gentle relationship with myself. This would decrease my self-intimacy and make it impossible to be intimate with others. If I am going to accept the reality that I, Darrin Ford, was raped, I must acknowledge that I have and will continue to have strong feelings of anger. This is completely normal. Feelings of anger will show themselves in many ways, and this is okay as well. Acceptance is not denying feelings; it is to consciously move closer to those feelings and see them for what they are, allowing the potency of the emotions to present themselves. If you allow that to happen long enough, you will gain emotional tolerance for them. You will possess the skillful wisdom to use that very painful and anger-provoking experience to help others. Why? Because you will have helped yourself.

Contrary to the mind's story, there are many gifts (and few burdens) of acceptance. The mind will say that having acceptance is overly difficult, and that acceptance leaves you flooded with emotions that you cannot handle. This is false. It is the mind's lack of acceptance of those emotional states that creates the struggle. If the mind says that having acceptance is overly difficult, it is proving that the mind lacks acceptance. There is no way around the reality that we feel. Emotions are not positive or negative; they just are.

People often find this difficult to accept, refusing to think of happiness as anything other than positive and anger as negative. This is a non-wise view of life. For example, think about unbridled joy (what therapists label as mania). When one believes that everything is and will be great no matter what is happening, they will produce negative behaviors—such as spending all their money in sprees or running into traffic without the awareness to pause for safety's sake. They will do this because the mind is assuring them that no matter what, all will be well. Unbridled joy, or mania, is one of the most difficult psychological disturbances to treat. Those who experience mania believe their mind's story that they don't need help. They don't want to change because the mind tells them that they are experiencing "positive emotions."

In reality, all emotions can be constructive and/or destructive. It is best to get to know what each of these emotions are like intimately. By doing so, we can identify them and glean their wisdom without impulsive reactivity. This can only be done if we accept these emotions and remember that all things in the universe are transitory, including all emotional states.

Acceptance is mindful awareness—being fully present with someone or something. With continued acceptance, we gain the serenity talked about in 12-step programs. In Buddhist thought, this is called nirvana. Regardless, it is not some magical, mythical place we get to. It is an honest, love-abiding acceptance of what is right here and now, nothing more or less; that is the true gift of acceptance.

Exercise: The Four Commitments

Being gentle with yourself encompasses a minimum of four specific commitments:

1. Practice the idea of doing no harm. This will be discussed in the metta chapter.

2. Practice the idea of not using intoxicating substances. This will be discussed in the awareness chapter.

3. Practice the idea of not lying/stealing, which we refer to as speaking unwisely. —This will be discussed in the honesty chapter.

4. Practice healthy sex and sexuality. This will be discussed in the sex chapter.

Each of these four ideals are not absolutes; they are constants, daily practices we do to gain the ability to connect with ourselves. In order to connect to ourselves, we need to know some things about the mind and the process of meditation. With some background on these two things, we can look more closely at these four commitments.

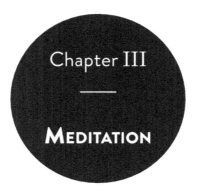

Chapter III

MEDITATION

"If you meet the Buddha on the road, kill him."
-LÍNJÌ YÌXUÁN

The day was warm when I finally built up the courage to go to the Shambhala Center in Los Angeles, California. I was immediately shocked; after the hurried and noisy street, I found myself in a still, quiet space that confused my senses. I removed my shoes and stepped onto a light brown, soft carpet, which soothed and comforted my bare feet. As I moved through the first room, I gazed at Buddhist statues and colorful illustrations on the wall. To my left was a small kitchen, and before me was a doorway that opened into a large meditation room. A hardwood floor and several red zafus were lined five wide and seven deep. At the front of the room was a raised platform with an oversized cushion and a large brass bowl with a wooden stick inside of it. The walls were white with windows on each side.

A friendly man walked out and introduced himself. He took me to one of the zafus and asked, "Have you meditated before?"

"No, this is my first time. My therapist encouraged me to begin practicing meditation."

"That's how I got started." He smiled and proceeded to give me some basic instruction, informing me that the formal meditation would begin in five minutes. I was eager, so I went to the front and grabbed a cushion. The clock ticked, the ceiling fans whirled, and people began to fill the room until finally, an older woman, who turned out to be the meditation instructor, arrived. She went to the raised platform, sat on the oversized cushion, and said absolutely nothing.

She sat in perfect silence as the fan whirled. I became increasingly unsettled. My mind reacted in fear and did what all minds do—it made hypotheses about how I must have missed something. It told me a story that all these people knew something that I didn't. "See, you should not be here. You don't know what the hell you are doing!"

With my awareness snagged by such thoughts, my anxiety and fear swelled. The loudness of my self-doubt grew until it was cut off by the ringing of the brass meditation bowl.

It hummed loudly throughout the room, clearing my mind unexpectedly, much like ginger clears the palate of wasabi. When the sound faded to nothing, she finally spoke, talking for just a few moments. Then, she asked the audience if there were any questions before we started our official sit. To my dismay, there were no questions.

"Start the sit," she said. My fear spiked, and my mind's stories elaborated: They are all so calm. You are not calm. They are calm. You cannot do this. This is never going to work, and now, because you sat at the front, you cannot leave. If you get up now, everyone will watch you. You are stuck, and yet, you cannot do this meditation thing.

I raised my hand. By this time, my right knee was bouncing nervously. In a loving, calm, and gentle voice, the teacher asked what my question was. I responded with, "I am not sure if it is a question or more of a statement. I mean, I don't think I can do this… no, no, I know I cannot do this. I am just here right now and have not even started the meditation, and I can hardly sit here." I was rambling.

Because I was in the front row, she was very close to me, just slightly elevated on the platform. She leaned forward and asked, "What is your name?"

"Darrin," I replied.

My right knee was vibrating up and down. She reached out with her hand and lightly placed it on my knee. My body froze. In a subtle, compassionate voice, she said, "Darrin, I want you to know that I am not sure of very many things in this world, but one thing I know for sure is nobody has ever died from meditation. You are going to be okay."

At that moment, my mind's story was exposed. I laughed. The room was filled with compassionate and joyful energy. I agreed with her. Then, she realized her posture, asked us to notice ours, and rang the bowl again. I sat the entire time in silence. I did not die. That day I began the single most powerful practice I have ever participated in.

I was addicted to meditation after that first sit. During certain periods in my life, I would practice each day, sometimes entire weekends. Other periods, I walked away from the practice, only to return. To this day, I have such gratitude for that moment. Whenever my fears get the best of me, I place my hand on my knee and remind myself that no one has ever died from meditation, and I will be okay. This practice may be hard for you at the beginning, as it was for me. You too, will, and can do this. All you need is consistency, practice, and compassion. Meditation practice is just that—a practice.

Each meditation should be done in a quiet environment. Make an effort to avoid interruption. Create a safe, quiet space for yourself. It does not need to be in your home.

Many times, I will meditate in my car. After lunch, I will practice in my office. Everyone there knows that from 1–2 p.m., if the lights are out, I am in meditation. Now, I won't lie; sometimes that hour becomes a siesta, and that is okay. I always tell people that if you fall asleep during meditation, your body is telling you that more sleep is needed.

You don't need a ritualistic place to meditate. You simply need a quiet place where you can allow yourself to sit, lie, stand, or even walk. Yes, you can perform meditation while sitting, standing, walking, and lying down. I recommend using a meditation timer app on your device. Most are free and easy to use. Just be sure to silence the rest of your device.

For the first week of your mindfulness practice, start with five minutes per session. If you wish to do more, that is fine. Sometimes, people are unable to do five minutes, and that is okay. If you end up doing 30 seconds, that is also okay. Remember that this is a practice, and over time, it gets easier.

How do we make time to meditate?

There is a wonderful podcast called *Buddhist Geeks* that I listen to, and on one particular episode, a guest used the acronym RPM to talk about his meditation schedule, which stuck with me:

- R = Rise
- P = Pee

- M = Meditate

I am sure your mind is screaming all types of stories right now, so let's just put something out there: you do have time to meditate, but you don't realize you do! You'll be amazed—the more time you spend meditating, the more you realize how much time you have to do so.

Let's break this down: How much time have you spent in active addiction? You know the work it takes to engage your drug or behavior of choice—the searching, traveling, funding, and hiding; the time spent intoxicated or engaging in behaviors; the time it takes to physically and mentally recover from the engagement. It all adds up to a tremendous amount of time and resources.

If you had time to act out in any form of active addiction, you have time to meditate. If you watch the news in the morning while having your coffee, turn it off. Drink your coffee next to a window; the morning is a wonderful time to meditate. If you can create a more formal meditation space, do it. Make this your focus.

Red street lights are great opportunities for a reflective moment. I have the eco-setting activated in my car, and when I come to a stoplight, the engine turns off. The silence is a wonderful opening to notice my breath. Red lights used to be stressful for me. I now pine for them and their momentary meditational respites.

You can also give yourself one minute when you get into the car. Put the keys in your lap and notice your breath before starting the engine. Another great opportunity to meditate is just before bed. When you lie down to sleep, practice it then. No one falls asleep the moment their head hits the pillow. In fact, most of my clients tell me that before they started working with me, they had great difficulty sleeping. Many have reported discontinuing their sleep medications after meditating for some time in bed at night. Each of these meditative intervals—a moment here and there—can add up to a significant amount of time if we make it our focus.

I often tell my clients, "If I paid you one million dollars to find an hour to meditate each day for a year, would you?" Of course, they answer in the affirmative, to which I respond that their psychological well-being and their ability to have happiness, compassion, contentment, and calm in their lives are worth more than a million dollars. If you don't agree, observe the countless millionaires who seem emotionally miserable. I know my presentation here is harsh, but I don't mean it to be. As my dear colleague and friend Mari A. Lee, author and owner of Growth Counseling Center, says, "Consider this a gentle, but a firm reminder. You have the time" to meditate.

Eating Meditation:

To increase your awareness of taste, I encourage you to start with a raisin, a prune, or a grape. You can use any piece of food, but for the sake of simplicity, we will use a raisin. Take a single raisin out of its container and place it on a plate in front of you. Start with three deep cleansing breaths, in through the nose, holding the breath, then slowly exhaling through the mouth.

Now look closely at your raisin. Notice the wrinkles and color. Examine each aspect in detail. Notice how it sits on the plate. Notice how your stomach feels and what your mouth feels like as you think of eating it. Do you have an aversive response? Do you have a craving response?

After a few minutes, pick it up and feel what it is like to hold it between your fingers before resting it in the palm of your hand. What does it feel like? Slowly raise it to your mouth and place it on your tongue. Closing your mouth, do not chew it; just feel what is happening in your mouth as it sits there.

After some time, bite it between your teeth. What does it feel like to take a bite? What does it taste like? Mindfully chew, continuing to bite and chew. After some time, do you feel the urge to swallow? Don't. Keep chewing. What is that like? After a few minutes, swallow the raisin.

This may seem absurd to the mind, and that's okay. Trust that, over time, this will help you cultivate a greater awareness of reality. This entire activity should take you a minimum of ten minutes. You can practice this whenever you eat. At breakfast, lunch, or dinner, take the time to sit and chew.

Notice the sensations. Observe the food a bit before you eat. Write in a journal about what arises. Notice the differences in the process for you over time.

Noticing is vital—it is the tool we use to prevent ourselves from going into the impulsive responses that give rise to addiction. This is a practical way to strengthen the muscle of patience and distress tolerance. The act of noticing strengthens our ability to recognize thoughts before we act on those thoughts.

Body Meditation

To begin meditation of the body, sit in your comfortable meditation space, take a deep breath in through your nose, and hold it. Slowly let it out through your mouth. As you do this, notice the movement of your body and how the shoulders slowly move down towards the ground. Notice how the chest deflates as you exhale completely. Inhale again, taking in all the air you can and hold it. Slowly release the air, noticing the shoulders again moving towards the ground. Notice the diaphragm pushing the air out of the lungs.

Allow yourself to breathe regularly and draw your attention to your forehead. Notice what it feels like. You do not need to change anything about how it feels—just notice it. Is your forehead furrowed? Is it relaxed? Simply notice it. Then, come back to your breath and feel the air leaving the mouth. Do this two or three times.

Now move your awareness to the cheeks. Be curious about how they are feeling. Are they tensed or relaxed? Are they hot or cold? Keep your awareness on your cheeks for two or three breaths, and when ready, slowly move your focus down to the shoulders.

Continue this practice through the chest, tummy, pelvis, thighs, calves, feet, and even the toes.

When you have finished, I encourage you to journal what emotions arose as you did this activity and what feelings you have now. If you can consistently do this for three months, you can review your journal entries and see the difference in your reflections.

When you first start your practice, you may find that five minutes is all you can do, and that is okay. Like I said before, even thirty seconds is okay! After the first week, I suggest setting a goal time of ten minutes for your meditation (or double the amount of time from your first week). Increase your time each week so that by the end of three months, you could be meditating for thirty to forty-five minutes or more. However, any time spent meditating (even thirty seconds) is better than not meditating at all. The most important thing is to try and do this consistently. Practice it as if you were practicing the piano or learning to ride a bike. Practice is key.

WALKING MEDITATION

Walking meditation is not just a wonderful way to get your steps in—it is also good for the entire body and mind. For walking meditation, I recommend that you start with a series of different exercises to begin to focus the mind.

When we practiced body meditation, we moved our awareness from our head to our toes. With walking meditation, we move our awareness from our toes to our head.

Activity A: Beginner

Find a patch of grass or sand you can walk on. Remove your shoes and step onto the patch. Take three cleansing breaths and start your focus on your toes. Then move your awareness to the bottom of the feet. Eventually, move your awareness to the entirety of your feet. This process can sometimes take fifteen minutes just by itself.

Move your attention up to your ankle. Then slowly move your mind's focus up the leg to the calf, knee, thigh, pelvis, lower abdomen, mid and upper abdomen, chest, shoulders, arms, neck, chin, cheeks, eyes, forehead, and scalp.

Now lift your leg and feel the weight transfer. Feel how the body shifts. Move the raised foot forward, noticing which muscles tighten, and which loosen. Be aware of the bottom of your feet and slowly move your foot down to the ground, feeling what it's like when it touches the grass or sand. Repeat these steps with the opposite leg.

For this activity, it is not about walking large distances. The purpose is about attuning to and being very intimate with the subtle changes and differences in the body as you walk. Ideally, do this activity for one hour a day.

When you are finished, journal your thoughts.

Activity B: Intermediate

This activity may be done on grass or sand, with or without shoes, but if all you have nearby is pavement or asphalt, you should wear your shoes.

To start, stand up straight and take your three cleansing breaths. Focus your attention from your toes to your head, as in the previous activity. After this, begin to walk. With each step at a normal speed, notice the muscle, weight, and movements of the body. Pay attention to how the leg absorbs the weight every time you step forward. Notice how the bones and joints move from the toes to the knees to the hips. With each step, simply notice these. If the ground you are walking across changes texture or position, notice how it feels different and how the body moves differently in response to the change. Pay attention to your heartbeat and your rate of breathing. Simply notice.

CHAPTER 3: MEDITATION

As your walk continues, the mind may wander to different events or thoughts. This is okay; it is how the mind works. Simply note it, offer yourself a bit of compassion, and come back to the body. You should ideally aim for one hour of practice. However, any time spent is an accomplishment. Remember that some time is always better than no time.

Journal your thoughts.

Activity C: Advanced

Cardiovascular exercise has been shown to produce positive mental health effects, and when you pair that with the cultivation of awareness, it becomes an amazingly powerful and efficient tool for mindfulness. This activity involves running and follows the same format as the previous activities. You should stretch and warm up the body before beginning and be dressed in comfortable workout clothes. You could be at the gym on the treadmill or outside on the street or track. Leave your music at home.

Begin by taking three cleansing breaths, then start your run. Attune to your breathing—in and out, in and out. Bring the focus to the feet, then the knees, then the hips. Notice the shoulders and back. With each breath in, attune to your posture, and with each breath out, attune to the relaxation of your muscles while maintaining your posture. Breath, posture, relax, breath, posture, relax.

Continue this for as long as your conditioning will allow you to. If you take a break from running, continue the same mantra while you slowdown: breath, posture, relax. Remember, during this process, the mind will wander. That is perfectly okay. When you see that it has, offer yourself the gentle compassionate reminder to focus back to your mantra: breath, posture, relax.

Journal your thoughts.

Lying Meditation

During this activity, lie comfortably, preferably on your back. Keep your arms to the side and don't use a pillow. Allow yourself to lie flat. You may do this on any surface; however, if you vary surfaces, it is beneficial to notice the different sensations that arise from each one. Take your three cleansing breaths.

As you lie, notice the body and how it feels to lie flat. Bring your focus to the back of the head, then to the shoulders, and then to the back of the legs and heels. Next, bring your focus up from the foot to the toes, to the top of the feet, top of the legs, top of the hips, stomach, chest, shoulders, face, head and breath. The mind will wander off path, and it will have many stories regarding this practice. This is okay. Just notice these stories, and with that gentle reminder, bring the mind's focus back to the body.

Again, remember that the ideal length of time for this practice is one hour per day, but you do not need to get to one hour per day overnight. You simply need to be consistent and practice. Always remember, some time is better than no time.

Mindstate Awareness

The amount of states a mind goes through is incalculable. While in recovery, any permutation can be approached through the five main strategies discussed in this section. Over time, you will find some of these tools are more effective with certain mindstates than others. However, don't get hooked into thinking that only one tool will work for you while the others are useless. We may have difficulty learning a particular skill, but that does not mean it cannot be tremendously useful. Therefore, all of these skills and activities that should be practiced. The more methods in your toolbox, the better.

Every moment of your day is an opportunity to cultivate meditational practice about each mindstate. Each interaction you have with another human being or with yourself is a perfect chance to practice the following activities. These can be practiced formally or casually throughout your everyday routine.

Use formal meditation to identify mindstates and approach them with the curiosity of a child's mind. Children are always curious about things, and they approach their inquiries with a compassionate, gentle inquisitiveness.

Mindful awareness throughout your daily routine is just as important as a formal practice. When we were in our active addiction, we engaged in destructive behaviors daily. Therefore, we must engage in positive behaviors daily for recovery.

These are the five main strategies to face any difficult mindstate:

1. *Reflection*: When you notice thoughts arising, ask yourself, *what mindstate is reflective of these thoughts?* Once you know the answer, ask if the thought pattern is useful at this moment. If it is allowing you a bit of wisdom, thank your mind for that, and let the thought drift off like a cloud crossing the sky; or, vi-

sualize the thought as a piece of wood floating down the river, revealing its wisdom for a moment before the water removes it from our field of view. If the mindstate is not useful or constructive, still notice it drift off like that lovely floating piece of wood going down the river.

2. *Choosing an Antidote*: You are standing in line at the supermarket after a long day at work. The person in front of you is at the checkout register, and they are upset because the item they are buying has rung up for a higher cost than they expected. They argue with the clerk, and more people pile behind you in line. The clerk gets on the intercom and asks for a price check. As time ticks by, you feel anger. The mind fabricates harsh stories about the person in front of you.

Sound familiar? This is a perfect opportunity for you to become aware of the judgmental mindstate. There is no need to become judgmental of being judgmental. Simply say to yourself, *Breathe. It is okay. This is what the mind does. Thank you, mind, for allowing me to have awareness of this feeling of anger. It is a normal reaction and part of being human.*

Alternatively, you can wonder what this person's life is like. If you have the time and energy to cultivate anger towards this person, you have the time to offer them an antidote: loving compassion. You can go one step further and visualize a white light emanating from your heart and moving towards the person. You can visualize this light moving towards the clerk as well, now that you see he is equally stressed. You are now offering loving compassion in your mind's eye to two people who you felt angry and judgmental at a minute ago. Let them know you are fine. Smile at them.

If you rolled your eyes just now, ask yourself: what emotion would you rather feel: anger or loving compassion? This is an important question to ponder because the relationship between thoughts and emotions are that emotions create thoughts, and those thoughts will reciprocally fuel the response. If we latch onto anger and judgment, they will be elevated in you. What would you rather increase: anger and judgment or compassion and love? Whichever we choose will be stronger within us. Remember that feelings become thoughts that turn into beliefs, which fuel behaviors into habits that then drive your destiny. Therefore, we need to be skillful with how we apply the focus of the mind.

Note that you should also be careful not to suppress your emotions. If you are feeling anger, shame, guilt, pain, or any other emotions that the mind enjoys labeling as distressing, our goal is not to deny its existence. Our goal is simply to ask: what is the most skillful response to the emotion we are experiencing? The emotion is then acknowledged and felt in your body. Notice how it feels, then begin to focus the mind on ways to have a compassionate connection with the environment around you.

3. *Scrutinizing Thoughts.* If you are experiencing a compulsive mindstate, remind yourself of the impermanence of all things. Offer yourself loving compassion as you take note of your mindstate. Sit with your urge, whatever it may be.

Look around the room and pick an object. Ask yourself, how long will it take for this item to disintegrate? You can even remind yourself that it is in the process of disintegration, moving from order to disarray as you are observing it. Your sense organs cannot tell that it is, but just like everything, it is disintegrating.

As they say in 12-step meetings, *play the tape all the way through*. Ask yourself, "If I allow awareness to get hooked into this compulsive mindstate, where will it take me? If I participate in this behavior, what will the outcome be? Will I feel joy? Will I feel shame?"

Investigate the outcomes. Write down a dialogue with your craving or compulsive mind. Ask these questions, then respond to them.

4. *Attention Realignment.* If your aversive, compulsive, or delusional mindstate persists, recognize the thoughts and move your attention towards your environment. Listen to the sounds around you like the blowing wind or the clickity-clack of a coworker's keyboard. If noticing environmental sounds does not work, utilize the skills you have been practicing in meditation—come back to your breath. Say to yourself, "There are those thoughts, now back to my breath."

The concept is simple to describe but difficult to execute. With practice, it becomes a great way to prevent one's awareness from being hooked by the unskillful mindstate.

5. *Remove Yourself from the Trigger.* Another intervention to utilize on difficult mindstates is to remove the trigger of these states by immersing yourself in a completely different environment.

Recognize that you are beginning to be flooded with a mindstate that is pushing unskillful thoughts or behaviors. Look at the environment you are in and respond in a skillful manner. By removing yourself from the environment, you may be able to reach out for help. The psychologist Dr. Tara Brach has a great acronym for this—RAIN:

- R = Recognize what is going on.
- A = Allow the experience to be there.
- I = Investigate with kindness.
- N = Natural awareness.

Certain mindstates are overwhelming at times, even when we notice them, so it is important to learn a breadth of techniques. SOBER is another acronym we can use, which comes from the Mindfulness Based Relapse Prevention workbook authored by Bowen, Chawla, and Marlatt:

- S = Stop.
- O = Observe.
- B = Breathe.
- E = Evaluate.
- R = Respond, mindfully.

Next to *evaluate*, I would add that you should do so with an open mind and an open heart.

Gratitude

The sun radiated from the pavement of the 105 freeway as an ocean of cars from every direction stood completely still. It was 3 p.m. on the last day of April in 1998, and I was heading to work at the Los Angeles International Airport. After sitting still on the freeway for twenty minutes, I knew that I would not be making it on time. The person on the road next to me made the best of the situation—he was sunbathing on the hood of his car. People had casually exited their vehicles and formed little chat groups. The question was, why were we stopped?

I turned on National Public Radio to see if I could glean any information. I learned that the reason for the traffic jam was a man named Daniel V. Jones from Long Beach, California. He was forty years old and drove a small gray truck with his companion, Gladdis, a Labrador whippet who was riding shotgun. He parked his truck on the transition loop that connected the Harbor and Century freeways. Police responded to calls from motorists who informed them that a man had parked on the freeway and was waving a gun around. In no time, news helicopters and police formed around the perimeter. Daniel unveiled a black banner with white lettering that read, "HMOs are only in it for the money!! Live free, love safe, or die." He returned to the cab of his truck and phoned 911. He spoke incoherently, making little sense to the operator.

Chapter 3: Meditation

What no one knew at the time was that Daniel had been diagnosed with HIV and recently diagnosed with having a tumor on his neck. His HMO insurance was not responding in a fashion that Daniel wanted or needed them to. These were the events that drove this man to his breaking point.

Despite the police's attempts at negotiating with him, Daniel set his truck ablaze with a Molotov cocktail and ended his life with a shotgun. News cameras and motorists watched it all unfold. Everyone on this day was pained, but not as much as Daniel.

I turned off my radio. The time ticked on. The police would not allow traffic to flow until everything was deemed safe. The Century Freeway is unique in that the Green Line Metro ran down the middle of it. As I was in the far-left lane, closest to the docking station, I was able to hear the Metro announcer give updates. At one point, the announcer stated that the train service would resume shortly. As he was speaking, he made a slip of the tongue that has stuck with me to this day: "I would like to thank you all for the inconvenience." He paused before correcting himself: "I meant to say, I thank you all for your patience, and I am sorry for the inconvenience."

The phrase, "Thank you for the inconvenience," affected me, and it is something I have used and repeated to myself many times. I find it especially helpful when my mind is trapped in a terrible and awful state. I take a deep breath and say, "Thank you for the inconvenience." Then I think of

Daniel and the love that he needed. I think about how the distress that I am feeling is nothing more than an inner part of myself in need of love, like that part of Daniel who was reaching out (in a horrific way) for someone to show him how to love himself. He needed anyone, including the system, to love him in a way he had not learned how to. I thank Daniel in my mind, tell him how sorry I am for his pain, and I offer myself loving compassion, reminding myself that if it was not for that day when I was stopped on the freeway, in a situation that was called an "inconvenience," I would not have learned how to see the need we all have for loving compassion in our lives.

I use the memory of Daniel to push myself to love more, to be gentler, and most of all, to have gratitude for each moment of my life. This is the power of gratitude. When the mind plays havoc with you and tells you that the turbulence of life is impossible and too difficult to manage—stop, breathe, and offer yourself loving compassion. In a calm abiding way, step forward into the unknown in an inquisitive and kind manner. For it is only with gratitude, compassion, gentleness, and a willingness to embrace the discomfort that we can discover those hidden and hurt parts of ourselves and then offer them the love and belonging Daniel so needed. Thank you, Daniel. I will never know more about you than what I have shared here, but you will always be held in my heart. You will always be loved. Thank you for helping me learn to love more deeply, both others and myself.

There are many lessons we can learn from Daniel's story. Another lesson that I have learned is how a mind robbed of compassion can lead us to very dark, desperate, and reactive behaviors. Had he been able to foster compassion for himself, or had our society been able to foster compassion for him, he would have been able to *cultivate a culture* of support. A culture of support is a community that shows compassion to your humanity. Cultivating this culture is paramount to a balanced way of living. When we are unable to have a culture of support, we may become flooded and overwhelmed with the struggles in life. To foster a community of support you must first become compassionate with yourself.

Remember that compassion is a verb. It is a skill and a muscle that must be exercised, just like meditation. We know from neuropsychology that the brain knows no difference between thinking about chocolate and eating chocolate—the same neurons fire in both situations. When we meditate on offering compassion, we are in the process of developing and strengthening the neurological pathways related to our ability to be compassionate.

There are various meditational activities designed to assist with this process. I have included a few here. It cannot be stressed enough that these practices are developed over a lifetime. To set yourself up for success, I recommend beginning with the first activity and work your way to advanced.

COMPASSION FOCUSED MEDITATION

Beginner

During this practice, begin in a quiet, comfortable place where you know you will not be interrupted. This meditational practice will take a minimum of twenty minutes. If you are unable to dedicate that amount of time to the activity, I encourage you to wait until you are able to do so.

Close your eyes and take your three cleansing breaths. For the first five minutes, simply focus on your breath. If you catch yourself thinking, that is okay. Just label the thinking, then come back to your breath. After about five minutes, begin to visualize someone you care deeply for: a dear friend, a lover, someone you are close to and who you are on good terms with. As you have this in your mind, say to yourself,

May you have love,

may you have joy,

and may you be relieved from all suffering.

Continue to repeat this mantra to yourself while visualizing this person in your mind. After ten minutes, begin to focus back on your breath. For the last five minutes, bring your attention back to the room and open your eyes.

Most meditation timer apps will have the ability for you to set intervals. This way, you do not have to worry about tracking the passing of time. Let the app do this for you. I encourage you to do this three to four times per week for a minimum of six weeks before moving on to the intermediate level. Journal after each session. After six weeks, review your writing. Share your progress with a meditation partner, 12-step sponsor, or a certified Mindfulness-Based Addiction & Trauma Therapist (MBATT).

Intermediate

During this exercise, you will need a minimum of thirty minutes. Start in your quiet space, free from interruptions.

Sit comfortably and take your three cleansing breaths. For five minutes, notice your breathing. If you get caught up in a thought, that is okay. Just label the thinking and bring the focus back to your breath. After about five minutes, begin to visualize someone you are close to and are on good terms with. Repeat this mantra:

May you have love,

may you have joy,

and may you be free from suffering.

After about ten minutes, move your visualization to a person who is neutral to you. It can be someone you don't know well, or it can be someone you have no strong feelings about. Repeat the same mantra:

May you have love,

may you have joy,

and may you be free from suffering.

Continue for ten minutes. For the last interval, bring your focus back to your breath before opening your eyes.

Do this practice for a minimum of six more weeks. You can also extend the time if you please. There is no maximum time for any of these activities. Some practice these activities for decades.

As before, journal after each session and review your writing after six weeks. Share your progress with a meditation partner, a 12-step sponsor, or an MBATT therapist.

Advanced

For this activity, you will need a minimum of one hour. Sit in a comfortable position in an area that is quiet and free from interruption.

Take your three cleansing breaths, then bring the mind's focus to your breathing. If you notice the mind becoming distracted, acknowledge the thoughts and move your focus back to the breath. After five minutes, begin to repeat this mantra to yourself:

I am loved,

I have joy,

and I am free from suffering.

Say this for a minimum of ten minutes. Now, begin to visualize someone you are close to and on good terms with. See them in your mind's eye and repeat this mantra:

May you have love,

may you have joy,

may you be free from suffering.

Say this for ten minutes before moving on to visualize someone you feel neutral about. Repeat the same mantra for ten minutes:

May you have love,

may you have joy,

may you be free from suffering.

After a minimum of ten minutes, bring your visualization to someone you have highly aversive feelings about. For example, for a long time, I practiced visualizing one of the two people who raped me. You do not need to focus on someone who violated you, but over time you may (and I stress, may) want to. Until then, pick someone who you feel or felt betrayed by—a brother, mother, father, sister, an ex-husband, or ex-wife, a former best friend—anyone who you feel anger or pain towards. Then, begin to repeat the mantra:

May you have love,

may you have joy,

may you be free from suffering.

As you begin to do this, it will likely prove to be difficult. That is normal and natural. If you are unable to keep your focus on this person while repeating the mantra for the entire ten minutes, that is fine. Move your focus to the emotion you are feeling. Notice this and come back to your breath.

For the last section, bring your focus back to your breath. Then, slowly open your eyes and come back to the room.

Journal your experience and share it with a meditation partner, 12-step sponsor, or a certified MBATT therapist.

Before moving on, I encourage you to continue this practice for much longer than six weeks. I encourage practicing this for a minimum of one year before you move forward. If you can do this practice for at least two hours at a time, then you will be ready to move forward.

EXPERT COMPASSION MEDITATION

This next practice is known in Buddhism as *Tonglen*. This is the process of exchanging yourself for another. This is a practice that can significantly alter our relationship to the emotion of pain and improve our ability to sit with another in a compassionate manner. Learning to be present with our emotional pain is the key to compassion work. Our ability to sit with emotional pain, without shutting down by impulsively reacting to it, will allow us to be present with those who are in their hour of need. I must stress here a couple of things:

1. This is a practice that should be initiated with an experienced meditation teacher. If not, you should be in treatment with a therapist who is certified in Mindfulness-Based Addiction & Trauma Therapy. An MBATT therapist is someone who has not only

mastered this practice for themselves but has also gone through the rigorous training and evaluation to become experts in the management of the emotions that will arise out of Tonglen.

2. If you approach this practice with an over-attachment to the ego, you will have difficulty coping with the painful emotions that arise. To clarify, if you struggle with codependency or certain narcissistic tendencies, then it would be important to discuss your intention to practice Tonglen with your therapist, your 12-step sponsor, or your meditation community. This is a practice rooted in the reality that we are connected to that which is far greater than just our egoistic nature. This is why I recommend Tonglen as an advanced meditation practice.

When I was first starting to meditate, I would do this practice while in therapy with my clients. I would exchange myself and be a filter for their suffering. It did not take long before I was out on leave from work because my anxiety became so flooding that I manifested symptoms of agoraphobia and panic attacks. I ignored the warnings of my clinical supervisor, Sachiko Reece—a lesson I will not soon forget. So, learn from me. This is a wonderful and powerful practice. It will positively impact your life and the lives of those you love. However, take great care. Go slowly.

Do it in isolation. Share your experiences, journal your progress, and be gentle with yourself.

3. Allow yourself time. Do not begin this practice on a day when your schedule is full. Take time, even though the actual practice can be completed within sixty minutes. You will still need to attune to yourself throughout the day. I encourage you to do your Tonglen practice earlier in the day, then set aside fifteen to twenty minutes in the evening to do a mindfulness-based meditation to check in with yourself and see how you are doing.

Unlike other meditational activities, do not practice Tonglen every day. In the beginning, do it about once every two weeks. Then, over a period of six to eight weeks, you can increase the frequency and duration of the practice. After years, you may get to a point where you can do this in your mind for each and every person you meet. I am not there yet. I continue to practice, and maybe at some point in my life, I will be there.

The presentation here is based in the teachings presented by Pema Chödrön. In her teachings, she presents Tonglen in three stages:

- Self-focus
- Others that we know-focus

- All the universe/world-focus

To begin this practice, you will need a minimum of sixty minutes. Begin your sit in a quiet place that is comfortable and free of interruption. Start with three cleansing breaths. Then, begin mindfulness meditation. Notice the breath. Notice the chest rise and fall. If you notice awareness being caught in the stories of the mind, acknowledge these stories and come back to your breath.

After fifteen minutes, change your focus. Think of what is painful. As you feel the pain in your heart, breathe it in, and then breathe out compassion and love. Continue this process. Sometimes, I breathe in the darkness of the world and breathe out a wonderful white light. When you breathe in, do not think of this as a constricting act. Often, when the mind is connected to the ego, the mind will become panicked and attempt to sell our awareness on the idea that the heart's ability to absorb pain is limited. It is not—this is just a delusion of the mind. You must align with awareness when this happens.

Awareness is connected not just to this body, but also to all that is in the universe. Remember, at this very moment, all of the molecules, suns, black holes, galaxies, and everything else in the universe has to be exactly the way it is without any differences for this moment to be as it is. So, in awareness, the heart is as limitless as the universe.

You must align with the reality that breathing in the pain is good for you. The delusion of the mind is that it is bad for you. How can we verify this? We are able to see that breathing in the pain of "another" is good for them and if it is good for them, and there is no difference between them and us, then it is also good for us.

If the mind attempts to tell you this process is harmful to you, note that delusion and align with the vastness of the truth that is in your heart. If awareness becomes hooked in the delusion that it is somehow bad for you, then stop. Take time, and start again another day. This is not a failure. This is a practice.

Take time to journal and notate the emotions. Allow yourself to be present with them.

On a different day, begin again. Take a deep breath in—moving closer to the pain of others and your own—and breathe out love, giving equal time to the in-breath and the out-breath. If the mind begins to constrict and close, notate that and come back to the practice.

Whatever the darkness is that you are holding onto or that you see another holding onto, you must become the filter, allowing yourself to see the delusion—that we must move away from these emotions of pain, shame, guilt, and anger—is the root of all suffering. With practice, we stay with ourselves and open our hearts and minds to those situations we usually move away from. Instead of doing what we normally do, which is moving away from these emotions, we move closer to them. We do this without reacting. If we begin to have a reaction, we notice this reaction and focus back on being a filter. Continue this process for thirty minutes.

Then, bring your focus back to your body. If your body is restricted, note this and come back to your breath. At this time, you just notice your breath, and you are no longer a filter for the pain and suffering of the world. Instead, we are back to mindfulness meditation practice. Continue noticing the body, then move your focus back to the breath.

After fifteen minutes, open your eyes and come back to the room.

Journal, talk to others and pay attention over the next week. Do you notice differences in the way you interact with the world? Utilize the curiosity of a child's mind. As you go about your day, notice if you are gentler with your thoughts about others, or if you are harsher.

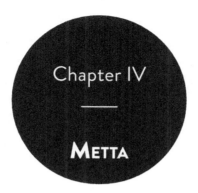

Chapter IV
Metta

THE PRACTICE OF DOING NO HARM

The sun was setting as nine men were getting comfortable in dark brown chairs. Stainless steel lamps emanated soft light just bright enough to allow each person to clearly see the face of another. Sitting next to me was a tall man who noticed a small gnat flying toward his arm. When I noticed the little guy, I felt a sudden sense of compassion. Here he was, with his small brain and body, attempting to navigate this room with nine giants who were causing (what to him would be) hurricane-force winds that were tossing him about uncontrollably. As this came rushing into my awareness, I saw the little guy land on the arm of the gentleman next to me. SMACK! That little guy was gone; his energy snuffed out; his world vanished.

Without thinking, I impulsively shrieked in what could only be interpreted as terror. My neighbor's face flashed with guilt and shame as he said, "Oh my god, I am so sorry! I forgot you're Buddhist."

I quickly thanked him and said it was fine.

At that moment, I became aware that I was connected to a lot more in the universe than I realized. It was a moment of awakening for me—I saw that the hours and years of mindfulness practice were moving me in the direction I had always wanted—towards the idea of doing no harm. In no way am I saying that you have to walk around watching everywhere you step in an effort not to hurt anything, although I have chosen to live my life that way. I am saying that if you want to learn to be gentle with yourself, then you must learn that when you participate in behaviors that are callus or aggressive towards others or yourself, you are not practicing compassion.

At each moment, we can choose aggression or compassion, but our humanity does not always permit us to choose the latter. This is why we call it a practice—choosing aggression or compassion a dozen times daily. Each time someone cuts us off in traffic, each time we wait in line, and each time we speak to a customer service representative who is unable to help us resolve whatever problem we are having, we have a choice. We either align with compassion, or we don't.

Choosing compassion puts us in the practice of recovery. The cultivation of recovery is all about learning how to treat ourselves and others in a non-harming manner. After all, there is no difference between them and us. We are all just trying to figure out this thing called life to the best of our abilities. If we practice the idea of doing no harm in the front of our minds on a daily basis, we will naturally increase our capacity for compassion towards others, including ourselves.

Millions of people have worked to gain sobriety. As we look at each program of recovery, we see this common theme: the idea of learning to not cause harm to yourself or others is vital to living your life in recovery. Every moment of every second of every day is an opportunity to practice this. We will never get it perfect. In some ways, we will always cause harm. When we do cause harm, we promptly take accountability by apologizing and taking steps to ensure we don't do it again. This is recovery—a lifelong practice of compassion, kindness, of doing no harm, and learning to tolerate distress.

If we are to reprogram the mind as it relates to our emotional states, we must connect to each state with care. When the mind has an aversive reaction to an emotional state, we need to produce compassion for it in order to form a new relationship with the emotion. Many in the West think of compassion as a noun; however, this belief is misled—I'm using compassion as a verb, an action. When I say we need to produce compassion, I am saying we need to act gently.

The relationship between mind, loving kindness, and compassion is simple. As you saw in chapter two, mind is a malleable, trainable, and organizing sense organ. The other organs send data to the mind, which then organizes and coordinates the input received. Mind draws on memories and emotional imprinting to formulate a hypothesis about what is currently happening, and it will project the possible outcomes of a given choice in the current situation. However, if certain decisions have been habituated, like when you're in your addiction, then referencing negative or positive outcomes for that given choice won't happen; the mind will simply react to the situation impulsively.

This is where compassion comes in. We have built a habit of impulsively reacting to our emotions in addictive ways. If we want to not act impulsively, we must build the habit of acting gently with ourselves. We must not believe the mind's story that we are somehow broken. We must realize that we are having a natural reaction to unnatural situations. It is not natural or normal for a child to see his mother beaten with a telephone receiver, nor is it normal for a child to see his stepmother have her face spit on and punched by his father.

It is, however, natural and normal for a child, who has experienced any type of trauma, to psychologically separate/defend themselves from it. This is what needs to be done for the child to survive. We see this repeatedly in trauma survivors and combat veterans. This is why addiction rates skyrocket for those who have experienced trauma, both emotional and physical.

Trauma can originate from a single powerful event, multiple medium-grade events, or numerous low-level events over a sustained amount of time. For example, incidences of neglect may not be highly intense, but over an extended period, the impact could equal that of an intensely traumatic episode. The effect is still the same—the mind cuts off from the emotion in order to survive, and if no one teaches that to a traumatized person, they continue utilizing that coping skill in all areas of their life, allowing addiction to flourish.

We must realize that we are not broken as addicts. We are nothing more than survivors. What we did to survive those events, which seemed so out of control, worked for us in the past. Now, we are in a different situation, and those coping skills won't work anymore. The side effect of using them is too catastrophic. It is only by having compassion that we can reprogram ourselves to accept the fact that we need to depend on those who can care for us. As those in our recovery community offer us support, the mind accumulates compassion—or what Buddhists call *metta*. This will teach us to behave in more compassionate ways towards ourselves and others.

Hence, we gain trust and grow ever more intimate with ourselves. As a side effect, we begin to feel, and as this occurs, the emotions may overwhelm us. Again, we need to be compassionate with ourselves when this happens by remembering that recovery is a practice.

Gentleness

At the end of a therapy session, I tell my clients, "Be gentle with yourself." This often leaves them confused—especially when they are new—and they ask me what it means. After a few sessions, they report that they're still unsure of what it means. When they eventually grasp the concept, they usually say, "I am not sure if I know how to do that." After several months (sometimes years) of recovery practice, clients have a light bulb moment—they realize what it means to be gentle.

Tomo is of Japanese heritage but was born in the United States. When he first came to see me, he had recently graduated high school and was attempting to earn an associate degree. He found the idea of being gentle with himself difficult. Upon his first session, I instantly picked up on how terrified he felt. Most of the session was spent helping him fill out the intake paperwork. He was so unable to trust me that he was afraid to sign anything, and it was not because of a language barrier; he spoke and understood English perfectly. It took years of work to establish the trust needed to begin to foster attachment.

His story was one of the most difficult I ever bore witness to: as a child, his mother would beat him and his sister daily. His mother would hit him with objects like hot irons and stab him in the legs with pencils. He would spend long hours of the day hiding under dirty clothes in his closet. He was frequently left on the couch to fend for himself all day. He would simply urinate on the couch, and the acidity would eat into the fabric, exposing the coil springs. To express his anger, he would pour his milk and juice behind the TV set. His mother would never clean up after these tantrums, and maggots would grow out of the mess that he made. He had no reason to trust anyone at all, and these horrible conditions left Tomo feeling unlovable, resulting in an abrasive relationship with himself.

The side effects of these conditions were that every time he interacted with his mother, he would attempt to please her so that she would not beat him. To complicate things, his uncle repeatedly molested him. Due to his harsh experiences, he never learned to value his own needs and would only try to please others. As a result, self-care was nearly impossible, and when he engaged in healthy behaviors—like going to the gym—he would overdo it to the point of injury.

During our first year working together, all he could focus on were the needs of others. If he was going to be late or miss an appointment, he became flooded with fear to tell me. He wouldn't eat or go to the bathroom until all external obligations were met. At the beginning of our sessions, he would show up famished, deeply aggravated, and angry with himself. After exploring his feelings, I would find out that he had not eaten all day. "I had to make it to my appointments!" he would exclaim. Much of our first year was centered around teaching him that he can take the time to care for himself, even if it means being late—an idea that he found troubling.

Over the years, he continued on his courageous journey of learning to care for himself. His ability to set boundaries grew. He leaned into his emotional discomfort and got into an intimate relationship. He not only obtained his associate's degree, but he also transferred to a prestigious university to work on a bachelor's degree. I once told him that he was the most courageous person I have ever met, and I still hold that to be true.

What he has done, you must also do. You must learn how to set limits with yourself—learn to go to bed at a reasonable hour, learn to wake up on time to meditate, learn to feed your body nutritious food. All of these behaviors are expressions of self-love.

At first, self-love may not feel authentic for you. It may seem confusing. Being compassionate with yourself can start with, "faking it til you make it." It is a fact that you are lovable, and there is no way you can lie to yourself about that! If the mind is saying you are not lovable, that is a lie! Only over time will the conditioned response of the mind begin to change.

Lovability does not mean lack of accountability. Being lovable is holding yourself accountable for the choices you've made in life. However, accountability is in no way negative self-judgment. For example, these thoughts—it is hopeless, I am how I am, and it is never going to be different—is not accountability; it is delusion. These statements mean nothing will ever change, which we know is a fallacy of the mind since all things are in flux; nothing in the universe stays static. To say that you will never change is a lie.

Accountability is not self-shaming or judgment. It is about recognizing the lack of compassion you had for yourself and others and taking action to prevent non-compassionate behaviors from occurring again. At this moment, things are the way they are, and the sooner we accept these circumstances, the sooner we can align with reality. Only then can we lean into the uncertainty of each moment in a compassionate manner. When clients begin to do this, they come back to me with an understanding of the phrase, "Be gentle with yourself."

When we discuss gentleness in relation to oneself, we are referring to a shift in the state of mind where one can witness our own behavioral choices. We may not know why we have made these choices, but we start to see the powerful emotions that arise—pleasant and unpleasant—surrounding these choices. We notice a pattern between emotions and events. We acknowledge that the mind creates stories. We let ourselves feel emotions without ridicule or reaction. We identify our aggression or self-destructive behaviors. If we've engaged in one, instead of condemning ourselves for it, we work to have compassion for ourselves. We realize that it is not gentle to behave in unhealthy ways. All of these realizations and actions cultivate compassion. This is what it means to truly be gentle with oneself—to use every moment, thought, and behavior (whether positive, negative, or neutral)—to cultivate compassion.

I am truly privileged to witness this process in clients—to see them awaken.

Wisdom

"True wisdom comes to each of us when we realize how little we understand about life, ourselves, and the world around us."
-Socrates

The topic of wisdom is misunderstood in the West as we have associated wisdom to the ego. Common examples of this are the highly reactive and aggressive physician, or the all-knowing teacher who is terrified to admit they don't have an answer to a question. We can see it in the public figure who appears to be so wise to those around them but has an unquenchable and uncontrollable need to be liked. This unbridled effort to shore up the ego leads us to addiction. In Buddhist psychology and in recovery, wisdom is an understanding of the illusory nature of self. To truly understand the self, we must accept the idea that there is no self—that all phenomena we see around us is incomplete, impermanent—and not the self. If everything is incomplete, then everything everywhere, including our bodies, are in a process. Think about it: your body has trillions of cells interacting and changing proteins and enzymes. There is nothing permanent about it. It is an ongoing process of cellular interaction. This is proven—all things around us (including ourselves) are perpetually decaying. Depressing, right? To the ego, it is. However, when we see it through the eyes of awareness, we find that it's truly liberating.

Nothing is Everything

If you ask a person, "What is the past, the present, or the future?" many will say the present is all we have, but that is inaccurate. The moment you have an awareness of the present, it is just a memory. The brain takes 22 milliseconds to organize incoming data from other sense organs. You have recognized a moment that has already passed. The future is a calculation of the mind to estimate what will be in the next moment. Hypothesizing what comes next is not a real event. The moment of *now* is the unrecognized space between the thoughts of the past and the projection of the future—so it is nothing—yet it is also everything.

If you are confused or experiencing a strong visceral reaction, that is okay. This kind of reaction is usually what happens when the mind or ego feels threatened by the idea of nothingness. The idea of nothingness does not sit well with the ego; however, we are born from nothing, and when we die, we become nothing—because that is everything. This is the basis of Buddhism's Heart Sutra.

To bring it down to Earth—the idea of wisdom in Buddhist psychology and recovery is to be intimate with the illusory self—to look at all the parts of our humanity, and not hide from them. Wisdom is to bring those hidden parts into awareness—to embrace it and say, I love you in spite of the deep sense of shame, guilt, regret, and anger I have towards you. I can allow myself to feel those distressing emotions, and at the same time, I can hold that part of myself in loving arms.

This is what Carl Jung meant when he described the knowledge of our shadow side as being the greatest gift we can give our children. I would add that the greatest gift we can give the world is a loving, compassionate knowledge of our shadow side. To drive it home more poignantly, I would say that wisdom is inviting every part of yourself in—regardless of the judgments of your mind—and loving every part of yourself. To do so will give you the ability to have loving compassion for all things. Why? Because you have compassion for yourself. With this in place, you will show compassion for all things because there is no self and no other.

> *"What lies behind us and what lies before us are tiny matters compared to what lies within us."*
> –RALPH WALDO EMERSON

Forgetting Everything You Know

There is no one too stupid to understand the process of recovery. There are, however, many addicts who are too smart to stay in it. An old Chinese proverb illustrates this concept well: A young man visits a martial arts master and requests to be taught. The teacher sits him down and asks, "Why do you want to study?"

The prospective student responds, "I already know a lot about fighting. I am in great shape, and I am very flexible. I just need you to see what I can do and to tell others that you trained me. Then, I will be respected."

The Kung Fu master looked at his prospective student, sat in silence, and offered him tea. The boy accepted, and the master began to pour it into his cup. It quickly filled and began to overflow onto the tea tray. The boy exclaimed, "That's enough! It's full! Can't you see that?"

The master said nothing and continued to pour from the pot. The tea, spilling from the overflowing cup, quickly filled the tray and was now spilling onto the table. The boy jumped from his seat and yelled, "What's wrong with you, old man!? Are you crazy?"

At this point, the master put the teapot down and said to the boy, "A man who has a full cup can take no instruction, and therefore, could never be a student of mine. If you were to be my student, the first thing you must do is forget all you know. You must show up to every lesson, listen to what is said, and follow directions."

The boy, realizing the wisdom of the master's display, was humbled. He apologized for his arrogance, drank his entire teacup until it was empty and asked the master, "Would you please be kind enough to train a scared, lost boy who knows much but truly understands little?"

The kung fu master agreed and pledged to train the young student.

I share this story to illustrate that recovery has nothing to do with your current knowledge. You may have mastered how to survive in crisis, and you may even be a recovery counselor, but that does not serve you in recovery. You may know how to hide your addiction. You may know the differences between yourself and other addicts. You do not understand, however, that recovery is cultivating a greater level of intimacy with yourself and those around you. In addiction, you were skillful at hiding parts of yourself, whereas in recovery practice, you allow the hidden parts of yourself to be seen.

The Path of Recovery

You must be sober to begin the process of recovery; although sobriety is not recovery—it is a step on that path.

Without it, you cannot align with the reality of your life. You may have heard of the "dry drunk," which describes people who have managed to stop drinking but have not learned to live in recovery.

Another step in recovery is learning how to set and accept limits and boundaries for yourself and others. This is not a quick or easy process. You will make many errors in your attempts to get it right, and that is okay.

This brings us to another aspect of recovery—accepting the reality that you are human, and humans make mistakes. Perfection does not exist, and everything in existence is flawed.

Aside from making mistakes, humans feel, and there is no way around it. Feelings are not something to be cured, avoided, or even "gotten through." Feelings are a vital aspect of our humanity. They are the very thing that addiction has worked its whole life to get you to cure and avoid. The only thing gained when we numb ourselves to feelings is chaos.

Another step on the path to recovery is finding gratitude for the wonderful things in our lives while simultaneously cleaning up the chaos that our absence from that life has created. This involves learning to forgive and learning to say sorry. Note that forgiveness is not absolution; those we apologize to may forgive and still be angry as these things are not mutually exclusive; we can hold both in our awareness at once. Forgiving those who may have been abusive, mean, or hurtful does not mean we are not allowed to feel whatever arises when we think of them. We can forgive and still have the feelings that we have.

Recovery is no short path and cannot be done alone—not because you are broken—but because the causes and conditions of your life have programmed the mind to believe in delusions. When the mind learned these ideas, you were young and unable to control the people who came into your life—people you grew close to and depended on. As an adult, you can protect yourself by setting healthy boundaries, aligning with honesty, and continuing to take contrary action to what your mind tells you. Most importantly, you can accept direction from a trusted therapist and others who have been in recovery longer than you.

As they say in Narcotics Anonymous, how we recover is through honesty, open-mindedness, and willingness. (I would add an open heart.) There will be times in your recovery practice when you feel it's all too much, and you can't remember anything you have been practicing. When faced with this, remember to practice compassion and be gentle with yourself. Do not forget that you are starting a new way of realizing yourself and the world, all of which will take practice, compassion, gentleness, and wisdom.

Chapter 5

AWARENESS

The brakes on the bus squeaked loudly as it came to a full stop. Stepping out of the bus was like entering a steam oven; the heat was so intense, it was hard to see in front of me, and my lungs burned each time I inhaled. I crossed the road to get to work, located in a single-story concrete building on the outskirts of town. It was painted in gold shades with an Aztec warrior featured by the entrance, guarding the clinic. As I walked through the security gate into the air-conditioned lobby, I was able to breathe normally again.

I was starting a job as the administrator of a new methadone treatment center in San Antonio, Texas. Heroin addicts in withdrawal would commonly present themselves in the lobby, sometimes throwing up in the trash cans. Sometimes, we'd find a client unconscious in the bathroom, or we'd discover that the bathroom walls were sprayed with blood from a person trying to shoot up. It was a difficult job; I saw the world of heroin addiction up close and personal.

As I became less green, we established a protocol for these events and brought structure to the office. We scheduled weekly meetings, during which we would discuss the progress of our outreach, HIV-testing, and our methadone program. I would write ideas on the whiteboard, while my team took notes and offered suggestions.

As the months ticked by, we made great strides in the neighborhood, increasing the enrollment in our programs substantially. I continued to take that bus, the brakes continued to squeak, only now when I walked across that road, people greeted me: "Hey, it's the methadone wedo!"

During one of our weekly meetings, I noticed each team member backpedaling in their chairs as I spoke to them. Clearly, they were trying to distance themselves from me. I stopped the meeting and asked, "What is going on? Why are you all leaning back so far away?"

Silence. They were avoiding direct eye contact with me. Finally, Maria looked up and said, "Well, honestly, you seem very angry."

I was stunned but quickly responded, "What makes you think I am angry? I am not angry at all."

Maria explained that I had been yelling recently in these meetings, and they felt I was upset with them. They were too scared to come into my office to ask questions and were relying on each other to figure things out. As a result, rules and regulations were missed or misinterpreted, which I would then yell about in our weekly meetings.

I could not believe what I was hearing. How detached from my emotions I had become? I sat down and took several minutes to process what I had heard. I was totally disconnected from my team's reality, and I did not recognize my aggressive expression of anger. I had enough therapy at this point in my life to know that the expression of anger from my biological father was so rageful that I had a difficult time recognizing the aggressive expression of my own anger because, in comparison to my father's, I felt it was calm. For those who did not grow up in an angry environment, my "calm expression of anger felt quite the opposite. As I thought about this, my staff continued to stare at me. I took a deep breath, looked them in the eyes, and said, "I am so sorry."

I disclosed to them my past relationship with anger. I told them I would work to improve my awareness of all emotions. I asked them to always let me know if they sensed elevated anger from me, to help me become more mindful of it. Over time, it became a running joke in the office—my staff, who also knew I was a gay man, would say, "Oh look out! She's getting feisty!"

If we are going to live differently, we must [...] emotions and gain awareness of what is happ[ening in the] body when we feel a certain way. For example, w[hat are we] feeling when we get goose pimples, or when our stomach muscles tighten? Let's look at each emotion and the physical states that arise from them. We'll also review how that emotion is seen by society, how emotions impact recovery, and the gifts emotions bring if we attune to them.

ANGER

How Anger is Felt in the Body

Tension is frequently attributed to anger, especially in the shoulders. Clenching of stomach muscles, arms recoiling, and tightening of the jaw are also common. Body temperature can rise with the intensity of anger. As the emotion progresses, the shoulders will often move up and back—an evolutionary response called *posturing* that allows the chest to appear larger. Angry people often point, which is a watered-down version of striking a person or thing. Time speeds up, the mind's focus narrows, and speech and body movements turn impulsive. This is why it is important for us to take the time and space to notice the sensations and bodily responses that arise from anger.

Anger and Culture

Americans have a love-hate relationship with anger. Men are revered and rewarded for aggressiveness. We tell young soldiers they are heroes and send them to war. When they return to civil society with issues surrounding anger, we cast them aside and judge them. We elevate powerful people who exhibit aggression and anger—like Donald Trump and Steve Jobs—then condemn them when their volatile natures present themselves.

Western society has an elementary relationship with this emotion. For men, it is one of the only emotions we are allowed to express. We are told we must protect our family, yet we are rebuked for aggressiveness within the family. On the other hand, women in the West are chastised for anger. If a man stands up for himself, he is powerful, but if a woman does the same, she is hysterical. Because of these cultural beliefs, Westerners are not adapted to coping with or understanding anger.

How Anger Affects Recovery

Naturally, we experience internal and external anger as we cope with the wreckage of our past. I always hear addicts in recovery say that they do not understand why everyone is so upset at them, especially when they are doing everything they can to change. After all, shouldn't others be happy that they are no longer participating in the harmful acts that they used to do? These statements are often fueled by anger (and shame). If we are not aware of these emotions, they will lead us to relapse. Any anger that we are unconscious of may lead to impulsive responses, which are fertile ground for addictive behaviors since impulsivity is what addiction is all about. Therefore, we must be aware of, understand, and accept the anger we experience as part of being human.

We have reviewed the physical signs of anger. Now let's examine its expression in the mind. A mindset of *all or nothing* (also known as black-and-white thinking) is a sign of judgment. Having judgmental thoughts informs us that the mind is reacting to anger. Here, we can use mindful breathing to increase the tolerance of the distressful emotion, or we can reach out for help. If the mind can lead us down the road to relapse, awareness of the mind can direct us away from that road.

What do I mean when I say we can reach out for help? We can call someone in our recovery network, go to a meeting, or journal our thoughts. Reaching out for help does not come easy for many addicts, but with lifelong practice, the muscle for reaching out to others will strengthen. With time, consistency, and compassion, we become highly skilled at it. This is freeing.

Always remember that we can deal with our feelings, or the emotions will deal with us. Denying them, judging yourself for having them, or putting yourself down for experiencing them has not worked. If it had, we would not be struggling with addiction. We now must do things differently, no matter how distressing it may feel at the beginning.

Gifts of Anger

Anger presents us with many gifts. Without anger, we, as a species, would be extinct. Anger is vital for our survival. It provides focus, strength, motivation, and energy. It allows us to identify when our boundaries have been crossed, and it moves us to assert our boundaries. Anger protects those we love. Working in the methadone clinic in San Antonio, anger was the catalyst of a great awakening for me. I am forever grateful to my staff for calling out my expression of anger. I learned an increased awareness to my anger and my expression of it. I am grateful for my willingness to be vulnerable, and that I shared my experience with them.

FEAR

How Fear is Felt in the Body

Fear often arises in the stomach, upper chest, and throat—where suffocation and tightness are commonly reported. Multiple muscles tighten, blood vessels dilate, eyes widen, and nostrils flare, which allows us to take in more oxygen. Fear triggers the fight, flight, freeze, or fawn response. If the fight response is activated, fear converts to anger, and we behave aggressively. If the flight response takes over, we run. Freeze—as in paralyzed by fear or deer in the headlights—is an evolutionary response that leaves us in a state of assessment of the situation so that we might make the best choice possible for ourselves. The fawn response is a complex response to fear in which we work to ensure we please the person who is eliciting the fear in an effort to avoid our own fear. This is not about empathy for the other person. This is about placating the other. We end up taking on responsibilities that are not our own, and we sacrifice our own identity. An example of this is when I was a child, and my family would work extra hard to ensure the house was totally clean prior to my father coming home from work. We did this not out of empathy for him, but out of fear for our own safety.

Fear and Culture

There are many contradictory messages in our culture about fear. If we are fearful, we are weak; to be strong, we must be fearless. At the same time, we are condemned for behaving in ways that are deemed reckless. We are told we are weak and less than for feeling fear, but at the same time, we are labeled dumb or stupid for not recognizing harmful situations.

How Fear Affects Recovery

When we experience the delusion of addiction, our focus on the object of our desire is so sharp that we fail to notice the danger we place ourselves in. We are not attuned to the risk that is present when we have unprotected sex or when we score drugs. We also do not realize how fear affects our ability to ask for the help we need for recovery.

Gifts of Fear

I will illustrate the gift of fear with a story. On a cold November night, my partner and I were getting comfortable in our seats on the Airbus—a beautiful aircraft with a strong safety record, which I grew fond of during my days working at LAX. The plane is well-designed with modern amenities and comfortable seating. We were returning from Denver, where we had gone to support my sister, who was (and is) battling cancer.

The engines started up normally, and the plane began to accelerate down the runway. You could feel the bumps of the pavement as the wheels spun faster. Then, in a sudden and violent jolt, the brakes engaged. This was not normal, and you didn't need to be a seasoned traveler to know this. The plane skidded, dishes fell from the galley, and everyone gasped. When the plane came to a stop, a pilot explained that a sensor had been tripped. The plane's auto safety mechanism engaged, causing the brakes to activate. The pilot assured everyone the plane was fine, a routine inspection of the aircraft would take place, and when the wheels cooled down, we would attempt to take flight again.

A flight attendant passed by and asked if anyone would like a drink while we waited. Everyone raised their hands, except for us. The passengers were reacting to fear. Everyone wanted a drink to take the edge off. They did not want to feel the fear they were experiencing. We didn't want a drink, but my partner insisted we never fly Airbus again.

There are two lessons from this event: first, we all naturally feel fear when things like this happen. Second, the engineers had developed safety mechanisms to prevent accidents and injuries as a response to fear. If the sensor had not engaged and the brakes had not been applied, we may have ended up in disaster. Ironically, the fear we felt when the airplane suddenly braked helped us become aware of our fear. In evolutionary terms, those who fail to feel their fear become dinner.

If we can bear witness to our fear, we can use it to facilitate self-preservation. Through the awareness of fear, we gain wisdom and protection. We see this in everyday situations. Think of a car seat belt or anti-lock braking systems. Without the fear of accidents, they would not exist.

Passion

How Passion is Felt in the Body

Closely related to arousal, passion often lacks a lustful component but may be seen as appetite, energy, and excitement. The passionate person speaks at a quicker pace, with a slight fluctuation in the pitch of their voice, and a certain gleam in their eyes is noticeable. Their body posture is open, and they feel warmth in their stomachs.

Passion and Culture

Western culture often judges passion as positive, and it is overly associated with love, though they are different. Love encompasses a range of varying emotions, whereas passion itself is an emotion synonymous with intensity or enthusiasm. Lack of passion may leave a person with no direction in life. Conversely, finding passion in work or constructive hobbies can be a healthy expression of one's talent.

How Passion Affects Recovery

After hitting rock bottom and starting the process of change, the addict often becomes full of passion—a phenomenon referred to as a *honeymoon*. In the beginning, they are full of energy, running around from recovery activity to recovery activity. This is called the *pink cloud syndrome.* Because no feeling is final, the honeymoon will pass. The newly recovering addict must recognize this, for they may become resentful, and when there is resentment, chances of relapse are heightened. In recovery, we must recognize and be present with passion, and remind ourselves that there are many other emotions ahead, and all emotions, including passion, are fleeting.

Becoming passionate about others in recovery is a slippery slope since we are still learning how to be intimate with ourselves. It's tempting for the mind to be captivated with romantic passions for other people. This may prove a wonderful distraction from the difficulty of being intimate with the self.

Lustful passion related to arousal can be a beautiful way of connecting sexually. Unbridled passion, however, can move us into addictive and/or compulsive sexual behaviors. Even if we lack a diagnosis of sexual addiction, we must be mindful of this possibility; when we pull back on addictive behaviors in one area, they often manifest in places where they may not have before.

Gifts of Passion

Passion provides gratitude and energy for connection, and it fuels meaning and purpose in what we do. We use passion to behave in a caring manner towards ourselves and others, and we use it to share our talents with the world. Passion brings us closer to those around us and gives us an appreciation for this connection.

Joy

How Joy is Felt in the Body

Joy is a powerful emotion that manifests throughout the body; there is no one center for it. Contrary to popular belief, joy has a calming effect on our bodies. This misconception comes from mistaking joy for happiness. Whereas happiness is external and future-focused, joy arises out of vulnerability with the self. For example, people often say, *I'll be happy once I get that promotion,* or *I'll be happy when I'm married.* To have a moment of pure joy is to know your oneness with all things. It produces a feeling of lightness in the body that is all-encompassing. In my experience of deep meditation, I have attuned to joy beginning within the heart—where I felt it most intensely—as well as the upper chest. However, joy can be experienced in all areas of the body.

Joy and Culture

On top of mistaking joy for happiness, our culture demands that we emanate the latter at all times; if we don't, then something is wrong with us. Also, true joy can only arise out of gratitude, and our culture does not actively practice gratitude as we are disconnected from our passion and distant from vulnerability, with the ripple effect being detachment from joy.

In a moment of pure joy, we often cry. Think of the day your child was born or the time you awoke from your addictive mind and began to change the way you lived. In these moments, we are attuned to our vulnerability and to the reality that we are connected to causes and conditions far greater than we ever imagined. If we practice gratitude during these times, we will be embracing joy.

How Joy Affects Recovery

Most recovery programs include a disclosure process. Step 4 in most 12-step programs asks us to thoroughly examine character defects and assets, and make a list of amends that we need to carry out. Upon completion of the disclosure process, many of my clients report feeling light. What they are actually experiencing is joy. If they are in a relationship, this may be confusing as their partner is likely not experiencing joy. Their partner is often still hurt by the addict's actions.

The addict will then often say, "I don't understand—things are good now! I am not doing what I used to do."

The addict is not heartless, just perplexed. For the first time in a long while (or perhaps even in their life), they are experiencing an unfamiliar feeling called joy. In the meantime, their partner or family's anger adds another layer of confusion. The disconnect between the partner's anger and the addict's joy may provoke an aggressive or resentful mindset, creating a barrier to vulnerability. Their diminishing joy moves into anger and pain, the mind mistrusts the recovery process, and relapse appears certain. To combat this, gratitude should be practiced daily, or if needed, on an hourly basis.

After years of detachment from reality, finding gratitude (and joy) will be challenging. However, if an addict is able to go through this process and continue a mindful practice, they will eventually move into an immensely joyful life. Their joy will not stem from external things but originate from the relationship they have to their internal world.

Gratitude takes years of practice, but it does not mean it will be years before you experience any joy. The more gratitude you practice, the greater attunement you will have to the feeling. If you struggle to find joy, it is not because it doesn't exist in your life—it's because your ability to see and hold it in awareness needs strengthening. Each of us can find joy instantly. Just take a breath and attune to how lucky you are that you can practice gratitude, and how thankful you are to be right here in this moment.

Gifts of Joy

Joy affords us a sense of gratitude, and it brings us a sense of abundance and connection. It is often a byproduct of caring for ourselves and others through balanced, healthy behaviors. Joy is essential to recovery as it allows us to move into equanimity and serenity.

GUILT

How Guilt is Felt in the Body

Guilt is an emotion that manifests mainly in the gut and lower back. It presents as tightness in the abdomen and creates a slight excitatory response in the nervous system. Down-cast eyes, head bowed forward, and avoidant behavior are physical signs of guilt. The facial expressions are similar to shame, which will be discussed later.

Guilt and Culture

We cast guilt negatively in the West. A quick internet search on the emotion will produce many clips debasing it as useless, but there is no such thing as a useless emotion. All emotions carry vast wisdom if we attune to them. In collectivistic cultures(cultures that identify more with family than individuality), guilt is more readily accepted, written about, and discussed. In these cultures, guilt is less denied and more readily attuned.

In the West, guilt and shame are often confused with each other. To clarify, the former is focused on behavior, while the latter is focused on the self. Many addicts grapple with what guilt is because we lack the emotional sophistication to separate self from action. ddicts may believe taking responsibility is stating how bad and wrong we are.

How Guilt Affects Recovery

As stated above, guilt is NOT self-focused—it is behaviorally-focused. Guilt drives the desire to take corrective action while not being tied to defensiveness. Guilt is commonly reported when beginning a disclosure process; it serves as a catalyst for making amends. Conversely, the inability to process guilt can result in behaviors that violate our personal values and impedes attempts to make amends. For this reason, realizing the difference between guilt and shame would serve addicts in recovery because they can lean into the discomfort of guilt and take corrective steps.

The Gift of Guilt

Guilt allows us to experience a sense of containment—we contain destructive behaviors and gain humility. Guilt allows us to recognize our humanity. When we do this, we can make amends to others. Guilt is the key to being connected to the greater whole that is humankind.

SHAME

How Shame is Felt in the Body

Shame has been referred to as the dark messenger of the soul, and it presents itself in the body in a myriad of ways: the shoulders hunch, the chest closes, the eyes cast downward, and the lips tightly frown. It is felt primarily in the upper chest and face, and the latter often turns red. With guilt, there is still enough openness in the face to allow connection, but with shame, openness is not available.

Shame and Culture

In Western culture, people are driven by the attainment of more recognition, power, money, fame. While there is nothing wrong with this, the motivation behind our chase for more is often shame-driven. Every time we believe the mind's projection that we are not enough—not rich, smart, or good enough—we are experiencing shame.

We are greatly affected by shame in the West, yet we are mostly unconscious of it. Our inability to see and tolerate it is partially responsible for the isolation pattern we see in our culture today.

Our culture has become so detached from the feeling of shame that we do not recognize it until we are at rock bottom. We struggle because we cannot be present with it, which drives our reactionary ways with others. Whether we believe it's guns or people that kill people, behind the gun or person is our reactive relationship to shame—and that is what kills people. Shame does not drive us to react negatively towards others; it is our impulsive desire to react to shame. Our desire to behave in any way possible to numb ourselves to it causes these extreme behaviors. These behaviors crate intensity, which numbs us to the discomfort of shame temporarily.

Shame often shows itself as aggression and defensiveness. We always know unprocessed shame because it creates the desire to isolate. If we cannot connect to ourselves, we will never be able to connect to others, and if we cannot tolerate the discomfort of our shame, we will not be able to connect to ourselves.

How Shame Affects Recovery

Shame is the most important emotion for all of us, addict or not. For addicts, it's the beginning of recovery. What do I mean by this? The shame we feel after getting caught in our addiction—whether sexual, chemical, or behavioral—is what gets us into treatment, allowing us to pivot in our stubborn ways. Without the flood of this feeling, we would never stop doing what we are doing. Shame moves us into the action of learning how to be intimate with ourselves. Without the ability to tolerate the shame we feel, we cannot move forward into our guilt.

Many describe depression as being overwhelmed with pain, and this is true. However, as someone who has struggled with major depression for my entire life, I can tell you that a large amount of that depression was propped up by shame. Shame manifests when we deny our current difficulties. It is our mind's reaction to shame that creates those thoughts of "I will never get this" or "It's all hopeless" or "I am worse than everyone else." The truth is, you are NOT terminally unique. You, me, and every other addict are the same: we are human beings, and we are not special. We are having a natural reaction to the causes and conditions in our lives. As a result of our trauma, we cut ourselves off from our emotions. We spiraled out of control, unable to connect to those around us, unable to connect to ourselves.

Gifts of Shame

When we are in the darkest parts of our shame, we are forced to see just how violative our behaviors have been. The greatest gift we can ever give ourselves and society is the ability to sit with total presence in the face of our shame, to fully acknowledge how dark we can be. Then, we must offer love and compassion to that part of our soul. This is the first step in learning how to feel, and only by doing this can we begin to open up to all other emotions.

As with other emotions, the gift of shame brings us our humanity. If we do not have shame, we do not have connection. We must invite the shame in and simply be with it. We do not need to do anything with it except to let it in and know that the feeling will eventually subside—it will rise, crest, and fall like a wave. If you do not learn to be present with your shame, you and those around you will suffer greatly—for you will hide the most valuable parts of your humanity.

LOVE

How Love is Felt in the Body

Love is arguably the most misunderstood emotion. The physicality of love generally starts in the heart and moves throughout the body. Loss of ego and openness of the body are common attributes. Love is often mistaken for infatuation and/or arousal, but these are not the same things.

Love and Culture

We are naïve about love in the West. We propagate the false idea that somehow, love conquers all. In stories about love, the prince always rescues the princess, and these fairytale notions of love have damaged us collectively. Love rescues no one, and love does not redeem you. You do not need to look outside yourself for love.

Love is predominantly seen as positive in our culture, but just like other emotions, it can bring chaos and suffering. Without boundaries, it could even lead to death; there is nothing more destructive than unbridled love.

How Love Affects Recovery

We begin learning how to love ourselves when we are on the path of recovery. Self-love begins when we are present with the other emotions first. The prerequisite for love is compassion for ourselves, and to have that compassion, you must skillfully be present with all other emotions. Once we have honed the skill of presence, we can see the truth about ourselves—that we are, and have always been, loving beings.

Love is recovery. You may have believed you were loving yourself in active addiction, but you were simply avoiding distressing emotions. You lost the ability or were not allowed to love all parts of yourself in a healthy manner, which means you were unable to love all the parts of others.

Many addicts become upset when I present this idea to them. They will say, "But I love my spouse! I love my kids!"

This is a pivotal point in recovery. I compassionately ask, "Then why betray them? Why the lies and deception?" Love for a person does not fully happen without respect.

We could not love all of our partner because we were not able to love all of ourselves. When we rejected those parts of ourselves that were distressing, we rejected the distressing parts of our loved ones' psyche as well. We knew no other way. Our loved ones are hurt because they loved all the parts of us, and believed that you, the addict, had shown all the parts of yourself to them, when in fact, you had not. When this was discovered, they were pained deeply; they discovered they were in love with a fantasy that you had created for them.

Creating a fantasy for another is not love; it is a selfish act. Our mind tells us it's a caring act to protect them from hurt, but this is a delusion because it is really to protect ourselves from the shame we feel when we see them hurt.

Once we can tolerate the distressing aspects of other feelings, we allow all of ourselves to be seen. Similar to how the color black absorbs all other colors, the ability to feel love happens when all other emotions have been attuned to and absorbed. When we allow all of ourselves to be seen by those we value—regardless of whether they stay or leave—in that moment of showing all of ourselves, we have truly loved and were loved.

If your mind is like mine, it is screaming, "Wait—if they leave me, that means they did not love me!" This is not necessarily true. They are having a hard time too. Remember, the hardest thing to do in the world is to know we are worthy of the love another offers us. Our partners struggle with this concept too, which is why our partners need to be in therapy as well. An addict's relapse rate decreases when the partner is in therapy for themselves. We, as addicts, and our family, have been affected by addiction, and we must all learn how to allow ourselves to be loved. Only then can we fully embrace the love offered to us.

Gifts of Love

The gifts of love are a loss of egocentricity and the discovery that you are in union with everything around you. This may sound eccentric since we are fixated on love being about relationships. Relationships are romantic and manifest out of love—or, to be more accurate—connection manifests out of love. Connections can be romantic, spiritual, or bodily, to name a few, and all of these types reflect the gifts of love.

Even choosing environmentally-friendly products or services is a loving act.

Without compassion, there is no love. Underneath the process of recovery lies gentle, abiding compassion. We work to develop compassion as a tool that allows us to love fully and be fully loved.

Pain

How Pain is Felt in the Body

All of us are familiar with physical and emotional pain, both of which can be felt anywhere on the body. Interestingly, the same area of the brain—the anterior insula and the anterior cingulate cortex—is activated regardless of the kind of pain experienced. This implies that emotional and physical pain have more in common than we may realize.

Pain and Culture

"No pain, no gain" has been championed by the West for decades. If you stop to acknowledge pain, you are considered weak, unworthy, or somehow bad for doing so. The mythology of "no pain, no gain" is the same for both genders and crosses cultural borders. This is yet another source of our struggle to temper impulsiveness. We lose our ability to tolerate the discomfort of pain when we simply shove it aside as soon as it manifests. I do not mean that we should stop at the moment we feel pain, or that we should not work through it. We should, however, acknowledge it, lest we lose the wisdom or insight our pain was attempting to reveal.

How Pain Affects Recovery

Pain is the great equalizer, compelling addicts into recovery through the motive of having it cease. I often tell clients, "Pain is what got you here," and for that, we should be grateful. We must embrace each part of our humanity, no matter how painful that part may be. Of course, we have the choice to reject those parts, if we are willing to go where that leads. Whereas pain drives addicts into recovery, rejection of pain steers us into addiction, isolation, and oblivion. Embracing pain is easier said than done, but the alternative is to choose prolonged suffering.

Gifts of Pain

The drive to stop destructive behaviors is one of the gifts of emotional pain. It lets us know that we are behaving in ways that isolate us; it lets us know when we are connected to others. When we are away from loved ones, we feel pain from the activation of the same neural networks that are activated during the withdrawal from drugs.

Pain allows happiness to exist. This perplexes many of my clients. To illustrate the idea, I ask them for their favorite food (for myself, it's chocolate mousse cake). When they answer, I ask them how they know it's their favorite? Many provide a scientific response, discussing the concept of neurons firing, and when they are finished, I ask them, "But what does the mind have to do in order to know it is a good-tasting food?" Sometimes I offer a hint by asking, "What type of food do you hate?" (For me, it's liver.) And I ask, "How do you know this particular food you hate is terrible?" Commonly, they will say that it does not taste like their favorite food, to which I say, "Exactly!"

To know happiness, you must know sorrow, and to know love, you must know pain. One cannot exist without the other. We cry at a movie whether the ending is happy or sad as they are two sides of the same coin. The British poet Alfred Lord Tennyson summed it up best when he said, "Tis better to have loved and lost than never to have loved at all."

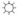

Having explored these emotions, let's return to the subject of awareness. To be in complete awareness would be to reach nirvana—to see without judgment, without forming conclusions, without actively influencing or inferring a thing, and to see attachment to what is seen. Awareness is neither good nor bad, and these judgments are traps of the mind. When we are not aware, we do not even realize it, and we suffer until one of two things happen: the pain is so great that we are moved into action, or our lives come to an end.

Awareness is not an observation for the purpose of conclusion. An observation includes the formulation of a story—one that you buy into to make an inference about the present moment—this is a distraction, not awareness. It is only when we watch the mind without buying into its story that we are in awareness. A wonderful example of this is when we find ourselves looking through the refrigerator for something to eat. Our mind may be telling us that we want food. However, if we take a moment and recognize that we are not actually physically hungry, we then have a choice to make. We can choose to eat because the mind says we want food, or we can take a moment and check in with the uncomfortable feeling driving the creation of this mind story.

We can be aware of anything if we choose to cultivate it. Everyone can become fully aware with sustained practice as it has no depth—it's not something that is just within us or outside of us; it's everywhere in everything we do if we choose to see it. Awareness empowers and can be cultivated in all states of being without the use of intoxicants.

Let's look at some examples of awareness.

AWARENESS OF FOOD

When you experience hunger pains, or when you know you are overly full, you are witnessing mind. Witnessing this process without judgment or reaction gains you greater awareness of food. You gain the ability to choose to eat or not to eat if you learn to witness yourself listening to the mind.

You will always have emotional and biological responses to food. When we are able to sit with the unease or the comfort that cascades from eating, we can become more selective with our eating habits. By moving closer to the discomfort we may feel surrounding food, we can begin to change our relationship to it. This assumes no limitations on our dietary intake. If we have an intolerance for a particular food substance, we will not be able to change these circumstances with only awareness.

THOUGHT AWARENESS: THE ABILITY TO SEE THOUGHTS

Thought awareness is not about reducing certain thoughts; it's about seeing all of them rising, cresting, and collapsing. At the end of the day, thoughts are nothing more than hypotheses about the past and the future, created by the mind.

A thought is a distraction from awareness, whereas to see a thought is a gift. So often in meditation, my patients will say, "I cannot do this. All I do is think."

I tell them, "This is great news." This means they see their thinking, and they notice their thoughts, which is what meditation is all about. It is not about the extinguishing or cultivating thoughts; it is simply about being aware of them—nothing more, nothing less—the byproduct of which is self-intimacy.

At the base of every thought lies non-verbal energy. We can think of non-verbal energy as unconscious energy or un-named emotional energy. Emotional awareness is the ability to attune to that energy. According to Buddhist psychology, cognitive processing happens in a series of steps:

1. Perception

2. Emotional Energy Rising

3. Thoughts → Beliefs → Behaviors

If we lack perception of our emotions, we lose the ability to be present with the emotional energy arising within. Again, we are human beings—we feel—and I drive that point home because we have been inundated by our culture to not feel. We are told not to cry and that being emotionally vulnerable is weak. But it's what we do with what we feel that makes all the difference. The less aware we are of our emotions, the greater power those emotions have over our lives; the less emotional awareness we have, the more out of control our behaviors become.

When my clients begin treatment at *Mindful Centers for Addiction and Trauma Therapy*, we start with identifying emotions, which is difficult since to identify one, we first have to attune to emotional energy. The first energies we gravitate toward are those that the mind has labeled undesirable. In psychology, we call this the negative bias of the mind. We tend to shift our focus toward potential harm—an evolutionary adaptation that has served its purpose. Distressing things appear on our radar first, so we avoid scary situations. This is why no one wants to go to a therapist—we pull people into distressing energies to get closer to their emotions. Clients always want to learn how *not* to feel certain emotions, to which I respond, "You came to the wrong place if you want me to teach you how not to feel. I am going to teach you the exact opposite. That's what you have not learned how to do. Avoiding emotions is the root of your disease."

People's need to avoid distressing emotions is also why we find a correlation with trauma and addictive disorders. The distress of emotions experienced as a child is too much for the developing brain to handle, so the child suppresses these emotions, works to move away from them, and relies on this coping mechanism throughout life. As an adult, they continue to find ways to suppress emotions. They lack awareness,

CHAPTER 5: AWARENESS

which ends in unfavorable situations, as illustrated in the following story:

I was working at an acute care psychiatric hospital in South Central Los Angeles for about a year, and I was about to meet up with Sasko, my clinical supervisor. She was an elderly Japanese woman who was formally trained in Jungian Psychology. As we began the normal process of reviewing each client, she quickly assessed that I was not my usual self. She inquired, "Are you okay? You seem a little off today." I explained I was tired, and that I had a disturbing dream the night before, which left me unable to go back to sleep. This piqued her attention. She told me to set my files down and tell her what it was about.

I dreamt I was in the waiting room of a psychiatric hospital when one of my clients walked through the door and collapsed onto the ground. I ran to her and found blood pouring from her arms. I applied pressure to her wrist and tried talking to her, but she was not responsive. I yelled for help, but no one came. Panic overcame me as I yelled louder, but no one appeared. I felt pain and sorrow as I contemplated my client's fate. I felt torn between needing to call 911, and letting go of her wrist, the latter of which would most certainly end in her death. I yelled in vain, "Help! Please, someone, help!"

After I told my story, Sasko had an intense look on her face, which was odd as she never seemed emotionally reactive about anything. She exclaimed, "You are in trouble! I want you to take the day off. And I want you to think about taking a vacation as soon as possible."

At the time, I was a hardcore cognitive behavioral type of guy, and I wasn't going to buy into the hocus pocus of Jungian therapy. I had no interest in the unconscious. For me, A+B=C, and I did what any know-it-all intern would do––I ignored her.

I had my first panic attack three weeks later during my lunch break. I went home and stayed there for six months, struggling with panic and agoraphobia. That was a difficult, unexpected setback, but from that point, I had a newfound appreciation for Sasko's knowledge and a growing admiration of the unconscious. If I had trusted her perception of reality over my own, I would have taken time-off, allowed myself to rest, and avoided six months of suffering.

In addiction, we are not aware of our own reality. We have no choice but to accept and trust in the awareness of those around us. This is the basic premise of surrendering in 12-step programs. One must be willing to accept the fact that they do not know and embrace the idea of trusting in those who may know better at this time in our lives. Put simply––we must allow ourselves to be cared for in a healthy way by others because we do not know yet how to care for ourselves healthily.

Chapter 6

HONESTY

"All things come out in the wash."
–BARBARA CANTERBURY

It was a cold, gray, mid-October night, and I had just completed my shift at the Gay and Lesbian Adolescent Social Services center. GLASS was a nationwide effort to help children and teens who were thrown out of their homes (or had to leave their homes) for simply being themselves. Though I found being of service rewarding, I was often left emotionally depleted.

When I got into my car, I looked down to see if my cell phone was still where I left it. I had received twenty-five missed calls and seven voice messages (these were the pre-texting days), mostly from Debbie, my sister, and a few from Joyce, my second stepmother. I knew something was wrong because Joyce never called me. Driving down La Brea Avenue, I phoned my sister, and she answered right away. "I have been trying to reach you. I have to tell you! I have to tell you!" She sounded upset.

I took a deep breath and asked her to stop talking. I knew that whatever she had to say, I could not hear it while driving. I pulled into a McDonald's parking lot, shut off my car, and asked her, "What's wrong?"

"Dad had a heart attack!"

The panic in her voice was strange, and at first, I thought she was overreacting. A heart attack is not good news, but it's manageable if medical attention is sought immediately. "What hospital is he at?"

"Darrin, he's dead."

Writing this, I still feel the sharp pain in my heart. I remember instantly beginning to cry. I had never felt pain like that before, and I had been through many rough patches by that time. I remember pushing my face and hand against the car window as I sobbed uncontrollably, unrelenting.

My father and I had our issues, but we had gotten to a point of mutual respect. He looked at me as an accomplished professional, and I looked at him as a kind-hearted person who had his own cross to bear. He did not have it easy in life. His father died when he was fifteen, and he was left to keep the house together. He was a narcissist, an alcoholic, and a sex addict. Those things were hard for me to deal with, but I have no doubt they were even harder for him.

Talking on the phone every day had been a recent development in our relationship before his passing. We did not sugarcoat our differences, and we would often debate over many issues. God knows it was hard for us to find anything to agree on except for two things: one is that whatever you do in life, do something that helps others not suffer. Two, no matter how much we did not like to hear what the other one had to say, we would be honest with each other. This second agreement was truly an amazing thing. My dad married three times and had multiple affairs. For most of my life, he lied to everyone around him. I was no angel, either. I struggled with my own addictions to drugs and sex. Two full-blown addicts coming to a point of complete honesty with one another was no small feat.

At his funeral, I remember telling people that my father and I fought often, but we loved one another deeply. I know today that it was that love that allowed us to be honest with each other. Honesty forces you to show all of yourself, not just those parts you think are acceptable. This was not an easy thing for me to do. I hid many parts of myself for years. My mind had this narrative in response to the emotional pain I was exposed to; my mind drove behaviors that distracted me from the pain I was experiencing. As a child, I lacked the capability to deal with the reality of my emotions. As an adult, prior to recovery, I lacked the awareness of my mind's defense mechanism of numbing my emotions.

That Which We Resist Persists

When we make that private deal with ourselves to hold something back, we are disconnecting ourselves from reality. We are cultivating an inability to be transparent. This process only builds upon itself, and we find ourselves alone.

Honesty is about seeing things as they are without judgment. Expressing facts with aggression or with a mindset that we know more than the other side is not honesty. This merely feeds ego; we are attempting to feel superior, which of course, is a delusion since we are not better than anyone, and no one is better than us; we are all human, adrift on a rock in an infinite vacuum called space.

Chapter 6: Honesty

Speaking Unwisely

Language is one of the earliest forms of technology, and arguably, the most powerful type existing today. When we think about language, we think of it as a way to communicate the inner parts of our minds with others—but this is only half of the equation. When we say something to another person, we send a message back to ourselves. When you point at someone, you point a single finger to them while three fingers point back to you. The messages we send others indicate much about the inner value we place on ourselves. When use speech unwisely, we damage ourselves and barricade our minds away from those who are close to us. We end up in isolation, coupled with an inner dialogue of unlovability.

When we repeatedly say that we "can't" or we "don't know," we gain a sense of learned helplessness. In 1967, Martin Seligman and other psychologists established the concept of learned helplessness from a two-part experiment that would meet strong opposition today. In the first part, three sets of dogs were strapped in place by harnesses. The first set of dogs were kept in their harnesses for a period of time, then released. The second and third groups of dogs were randomly electrified in their harnesses. The second group had a lever nearby that would turn off the electric shocks, which the dogs used successfully. The third group also had nearby levers, but theirs didn't stop the electric shocks.

In the second part of the experiment, all three sets of dogs were individually placed in a shuttle box apparatus, which was a chamber with a barrier down the middle, low enough for a dog to jump over. Psychologists would electrify half of the floor where the dogs stood. Dogs in the first and second group escaped the shocks by jumping over the barrier. Dogs in the third group did not try to escape the shocks. They laid down and whined as they were electrified.

This is learned helplessness—the absence of any hope that one can rescue themselves from their state of suffering. Once this happens, we acquiesce to whatever is going on, and we tell ourselves we deserve it because we are weak or bad. I tell my clients not to use these words. I remind them that they are the experts on themselves in the room. I am nothing more than a mirror that reflects back to them all of the things they say and show me through the use of their verbal and non-verbal language.

Why Do We Act Dishonestly?

According to evolutionary psychology, dishonesty arises out of the need to hide parts of one's self in order to survive, much like a chameleon changing colors to blend into its surroundings. Dishonesty starts in childhood, and I'll illustrate this with a personal story.

Growing up, I lived in a three-bedroom trailer with my mom, my sister, my cousins Tony and Jeff, and my aunt and uncle Karen and Ed. I remember each time the rain came to Mohave Valley, Arizona, we placed pans throughout the trailer, since the ceiling leaked.

I was nine years old, and my aunt Genie came to visit us. I had a cigarette in my hand when she walked through the door. I stood there with the cigarette behind my back. My aunt asked me what I was doing with a cigarette. I very sincerely and with a straight face responded, "What cigarette? I don't have a cigarette."

At that age, my only survival skill came from the primitive part of my brain, which told me to lie. Children who have been traumatized turn to this coping skill. They use it as they mature, and it becomes an unconscious habit, a go-to reflex during emotional distress. By being dishonest with those around us, we take a part of ourselves and hide it, which blocks vulnerability and leaves us isolated. Lies become habituated, and we lose track of what is and isn't true, what's authentic and what's fabricated. Real and myth fuse, all wrapped in a veil of shame, smashed deep into the darkest parts of our persona. Profound isolation, loneliness, pain, guilt, and shame are the products that flood us, allowing the addictive cycle to flourish.

Those who we love so dearly are left loving and knowing a myth, and when they see the truth, everything they know about you (and about themselves) falls into question. They lose trust in their own judgment, leaving them uncertain, fearful, and in need of healing. They need to mourn the illusion of who they thought you were, and they need to meet the person you are.

We can clarify mythology from the truth by using language wisely, and it starts with awareness of unwise language habits. Using language wisely will naturally develop from the practice of mindfulness. As we see our thoughts, we can strive to respond to others (and ourselves) without the impulsion to speak unwisely; we can choose different words and phrases, and we can ask ourselves about the implications of our choice of words.

Not Taking That Which Is Not Ours.

Though the concept is evident to many, others have lived a life where we (in some way, shape, or form) take that which is not ours. Culture, laws, and religion tell us not to steal, but when we are in active addiction, we do it anyway. We may have stolen to support our drug or sex habit, spending money that should have been spent on our kids, partners, parents, or any of our loved ones. Even if the money was not missed, it was nevertheless stealing and dishonest.

Aside from harming others, a more selfish reason not to steal exists: stealing interferes with knowing that we are worthy of love and is, therefore, an aggressive act to ourselves. We feel guilt and shame when we cause harm, and then we want to move away from emotional distress, like through addictive behaviors. We will pick fights with people because we feel guilt and shame and cannot resolve these feelings. That distress increases when we see them, and the mind focuses on ways to repress those distressing emotions.

My son was caught stealing from a local convenience store when he was in his teens. Even now, in his late twenties, he will not go into that store. I have encouraged him to, but he is not able to withstand the distress of his shame, so he avoids that place. Just as he avoids that store, we avoid our loved ones when we have been stealing from them due to the emotional distress that we cannot tolerate.

This is not limited to those we are close to or those we love. As with my son avoiding the convenient store, we can project our shame onto inanimate things or corporations. The antidote to this problem is to stop stealing and move your awareness into the shame. You can do this by disclosing what happened to a trusted individual like a sponsor or a therapist who can direct you on the right path to move further through these emotions.

When we start recovery, we are not remotely aware of all the financial, emotional, and relational vulnerability we have stolen from those we love, let alone from ourselves. We come to terms with the pain of lost time. During all those years in active addiction, we robbed ourselves of the opportunity to be seen and to heal. Each moment we acted out was a moment we stole from ourselves—opportunities to have loving, supportive, and close relationships.

When to Listen, When to Respond

If we have practiced mindfulness for some time, we can observe and be fully present when another is sharing. We communicate to be heard. If someone is sharing and you are focused on your own response, then you are not listening. Instead, you are in the ego. You are attempting to block what you may be feeling, as the other person is attempting to be heard.

When we listen to another speak, we hear their world and their wisdom. We connect with their hopes and fears on a level that is absent of ego; we are filled with emotional connection, and we change. We realize that their struggles and hopes are ours because we fear and long for the same things.

Honesty in Relationships

The addict holds deep shame, and the partner holds deep pain for staying with the addict. The former holds anger toward themselves, and the latter harbors anger towards the former. Both deeply fear the possibility of losing their relationship. When they share these emotions with each other, they are so reactionary to their own internal state that they are unable to hear anyone but themselves, which only widens the chasm between them.

In my practice, I assist partners in seeing that the very emotion they are trying to communicate is the same emotion the other is trying to communicate. I work to allow one to hear the other so that they both can also be heard. This is emotionally dysregulating for both parties, and I encourage each of them to seek individual therapy in addition to their couple's therapy. With an individual therapist, they can work to increase their tolerance of distress. They are each responsible for learning to work with sharp, edgy, and difficult emotions. Over time, with consistent practice, they discover that mindfully listening to each other results in a shift. The emotions that were driving them apart now connect them, which can only happen if both parties mindfully listen to the other—a process that first requires attuning to their own emotional energy and having the ability to sit with it, no matter how distressing. When we have learned to be emotionally intimate with ourselves, we open the doors to emotional intimacy with others.

People ask how they are supposed to do this, especially when they are being harassed by an angry partner. I stress here that we have the right to feel anything. We all have the right to be heard, but none of us have the right to be abusive. If someone is truly screaming, yelling, or acting aggressively toward us, it is our responsibility to set a boundary not just for ourselves, but also for our relationship. If this is happening, the conversation should temporarily cease until you and your partner can communicate without aggression.

When we mindfully listen to another, we can see their struggle for what it is, and we let go of our craving to control their feelings. We let go of our hate of their experience and embrace their expression with compassion and love. It is only then that we can connect. We have this opportunity every time someone speaks to us. We can practice this by wisely not speaking, and by mindfully listening to what they are saying.

Non-Verbal Speaking

The 747-400 was the largest commercial aircraft when it was first unveiled. Shortly thereafter, I found myself aboard one on a trip to Japan. Despite its size, typhoon-force winds jostled the craft. The rain pounded the window as I looked out into the night. The pilot came on the speaker and instructed the flight attendants to take their seats. The plane weaved side to side, teetering back and forth as we approached the runway of Tokyo International Airport. With each drop in altitude, the plane jerked and weaved with increasing violence. Then, with a powerful thud, the two back wheels of the plane slammed into the cement of the runway.

Having worked for an airline and flown quite a bit, I knew that landing during a storm was a terrible situation. Whenever a plane hits the runway, you expect to hear the powerful air brakes engage, and the sound travels loudly throughout the aircraft as you slow down. When the back tires hit the cement, I heard the engines rev instead, and I have never heard an engine rev louder in my life. We had missed the beginning of the runway, landing somewhere in the middle, and because of the storm, the pilot could not see this until he touched down. He immediately slammed the aircraft's engines to full power and aggressively maneuvered the plane upwards. Thank goodness for his decision, for had he not, our runway would have ended before we could safely come to a full stop.

On the second try, we landed safely.

Then, I rode an electromagnetic train to my destination—Fukuoka. During my ride, an announcement on the loudspeaker was made, naturally in Japanese, so I did not understand a word, but I did not need to. Everyone slid off their seats to crouch in the foot space, a nonverbal expression of fear on their faces. The blasted typhoon had caught up with us. The winds tossed the train mercilessly.

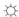

I learned much about nonverbal communication during my trip to Japan. I learned as much about effective listening as all my classes in psychology combined. Living in a country where I did not speak a word of the native language forced me to attune closely to body cues, all for a rudimentary understanding of basic communication. This was a gift to me as I gained much awareness, increasing my ability to attune to others.

Fifty-five percent of communication is nonverbal. We fail to take this into account when we are attempting to speak with others. Watching the shoulders, facial expressions, and what someone is doing with their hands and feet provides us with information. When someone is telling us that they agree on a point while simultaneously shaking their head side to side, we encounter mixed communication that leads to confusion.

Much of our body language is unconscious. For example, my clients may say, "What? I am not mad. Why do you think I'm mad?" As they say this, their voice is raised, their shoulders are moved back, and their eyebrows furrow. I say that I accept what they are telling me, but their body language is suggesting something different. They are stunned to realize how their body language contradicts what they are verbally stating.

Body language is most powerful when a parent is speaking to their child. To illustrate this, I ask clients to kneel as their partner stands in front of them, pointing and speaking loudly down at them. I ask the kneeling client what feelings arose for them. They are stunned at how vulnerable they felt when this was happening. By multiplying these feelings by a factor of five, they can understand how they felt as a child when their parents were upset with them. They can understand how their children feel at times.

I draw attention to this not to be judgmental, but to illuminate the importance of cultivating compassion-based awareness. It illustrates how the nonverbal communication we project affects others. If your nonverbal cues are aggressive, then regardless of what you are actually feeling inside, others will react to you with aggression or fear. They will be defensive toward you. In turn, this may leave you feeling agitated, and the cycle of isolation and separation will ensue. We must practice somatic mindfulness (body awareness) to increase our wisdom around what it is our body is communicating. We can do this through guided meditations that focus the mind on each part of the body.

I recommend a meditation approach called Mindfulness-Based Stress Reduction (MBSR), a practice founded by Professor Jon Kabat Zinn. The practice consists of noticing each part of your body, starting from your forehead, moving to shoulders and chest, down to stomach, legs, and toes. A few minutes can cultivate more awareness of the body, which will assist in acknowledging how others communicate with their bodies. The more we understand nonverbal cues, the more we will be in tune with honest communication.

Disclosure

Being honest with ourselves inevitably means being honest to those around us, no matter who it is. I strongly suggest not starting the disclosure process of recovery by yourself. I would encourage you to see a therapist certified in Mindfulness-Based Addiction & Trauma Therapy (MBATT) to complete a disclosure process. For sex addiction, I strongly suggest you see someone who is certified in Sex Addiction Therapy (CSAT) as well as MBATT. Therapists with these certifications are properly trained on the disclosure process. It is not fair to you or to your loved one to sit down and say, "Hey, here is my secret life that I have been totally hiding from you. Let me put this all in your lap. There you go. I feel so much better now!" without professional help. A partner will require support when learning of the dishonesty in a relationship.

Your 12-step meetings are NOT a professional therapeutic setting and should not be used as a venue for disclosing to your loved one. One should never disclose unless they and their partner or loved one are in treatment with an MBATT/CSAT therapist.

Eventually, there will come a time when the gift of pain will make disclosure necessary as you'll be tired of the doubts in your mind. After all, you cannot know if you are totally loved by someone if there are secret parts of yourself hidden from them. You have thought, "Sure they love me, but if they actually knew x, y, or z—they would leave me!" If your partner has asked for disclosure, you should provide it so that they can see with whom they are choosing to spend their life.

Your mind may be freaking out, yelling that there is no way you would ever tell your partner any of your secret life. Just remember, our minds got us into this painful situation.

Accept that you are not able to see things clearly and that your mind's eye is flawed. At the end of the day, recovery requires complete honesty, and that begins by living your life in reflection.

To begin:

- Get connected to others in recovery. Find a sponsor in a 12-step program.

- Get a therapist. Your mind will tell you that you don't need one, which is the very reason you do need to see one. Your mind will say it's expensive—in money and time—but what is the alternative? Living a life alone and in despair?

- Attend a professional psychotherapy group facilitated by a licensed therapist (preferably certified in MBATT and CSAT).

- Meditate. Sit in silence. Practice seeing your mind without reacting to it.

- Admit your humanity. We are not perfect, and we will lie impulsively, even when we are trying our hardest not to. That is okay. When we realize we did, we can go back to the people we've lied to and say we are sorry. We can let them know we are unable to see the impulsiveness in our minds but that we are working on it.

Remember that all of this takes time. You cannot change a mindset you have spent five, ten, fifteen, or even fifty-five years cultivating overnight. You are not broken, condemned in any way, or "terminally unique." There are millions of people throughout the world who have been right where you are, and through a consistent practice of these processes, they began to live a life that cultivated connection (recovery) instead of isolation (addiction), and it all begins with honesty.

Chapter 7

SEX

When I was seventeen years old, I was raped by a man who I had met at a bus station in San Diego, California. Being a young gay teen from a much smaller town, I was naïve to the idea of being gay. In my mind, I was the only male in the world who found other men attractive. When I was at the bus station, I saw a man who appeared to be in his mid to late thirties looking at me sexually, and it appealed to me. I was looking for someone to talk with, who I could show my closeted side to, but because I had grown up being molested by multiple people, I did not know how to ask for this properly. The only way I knew how to relate to another person was in a sexual manner. He attempted to have sex with me at the bus station restroom until he was interrupted by an employee. The man asked for my phone number, which I gave to him.

He drove from San Diego to my hometown—Needles—which was approximately a five hour drive. He rented a hotel room, told me to meet him there, and though I was flooded with fear and shame, I went in the hope that I would find acceptance from another person. When I entered the hotel room, he told me to undress. Though I was frightened, I did as instructed. I sat naked in a chair and said, "I don't want to do this."

He chuckled and replied, "Then why do you have an erection?"

I don't remember much after that question, except for having my face pushed down on the bed and the physical pain. I went home afterward, and he would call for the next several days in a row. He told me that he was coming to meet me again, and I told him I did not want that. He told me that if I did not meet with him again, he would show up at my high school and tell everyone what happened. If you can remember being a teenager, then you will remember that there is no possibility worse than being humiliated in front of your peers.

I told my parents what happened. I cried for a long time on my mom's shoulder. When the guy called our home again, my stepdad, Charlie, answered. In a clear, firm tone, he told him, "If you call or come by again, I will part your head from your shoulders."

I never heard from the man again. I felt so protected at that moment. My stepdad stood up for me in a way I did not know how to do for myself, and it changed my life.

As I told my sponsor this story, I was filled with rage for the man who had raped me, and I could feel the anger permeating from my every pore. The way I handled the anger—and am still handling it today—is not by denying it, not reacting to it, and not suppressing it. I allow it to be there; I allow the warmth of this anger and shame to wash over me. As I do, I remind myself that this is being human; anger is a natural reaction to being violated. I remind myself to be thankful that I can sit with these feelings today. Without this ability, I would be impulsively reacting to the feelings whenever they arose, which would be catastrophic as I would be back in my addiction.

Being gentle with myself means allowing myself to feel and accepting that part of human existence is feeling. Rejecting that reality would be an act of aggression toward myself. With gentleness, I can embrace all of my feelings, even when they are, at times, overwhelming.

As a younger man, I lacked the ability to do this. In fact, my brain was not developed enough to figure out how to do this. The unrealized shame and anger I carried were expressed in my life through hyper-sexuality—I saw everything in terms of sex, and the mind formulated that if someone did not want me sexually, then I was of no value to them.

In my twenties, I jumped from one relationship to the next with a singular focus: to have sex and to be wanted sexually. I was focused on my appearance, projecting sexuality, and gaining as much attention as possible. Living on the streets of West Hollywood, I would dance the night away at clubs and parties, priding myself on how many phone numbers I could collect by sunrise. At that time, there were no cell phones. People's numbers were written on scraps of paper, napkins, or my arms. I often wouldn't care about contacting these random people, but I would take the handful of numbers, look at them, and feel powerful and worthy.

Occasionally, a tempestuous relationship would spring up. If whoever I was dating ever said they did not feel like having sex, I would immediately feel worthless. It was as if someone had told me they never wanted to see me again. The unrealized shame, anger, and pain were overwhelming. I would react in one of two ways: I would leave them and find someone—anyone who wanted me sexually—or I would react with aggression. To discharge the unrealized energy, I would be verbally abusive to my partners. Needless to say, all of my early relationships were emotionally distant, and sex was the only focus. This is how my sexual addiction began.

To make matters worse, I could not accept my sexual behaviors because it violated my value system. My shame, anger, and pain boiled over. This could not continue, and my addictive mind found an answer in the sedative drug, Xanax. When that no longer worked to numb my feelings, I turned to opiates, allowing me to behave in sexual ways that continued crossing my values. My life became an unconscious cycle of sexual focus, lack of values, and ever-deepening shame, anger, and pain.

One day, I woke up in an emergency room, and the two fractured aspects of my personality had to acknowledge each other for the first time. The sexual abuse I had experienced led to over thirty years of disconnection. It distorted my view of myself and left me feeling empty. I saw other things, people, and places through a lens of sex and sexuality.

During that period, I had no other mindset to reference, but I knew that if I was to have a healthy relationship with sex and sexuality, I first had to have a healthy relationship with myself. The fact that I awoke in an emergency room after overdosing on drugs was clear, irrefutable, verifiable evidence that I was not connected to myself. This forced me to begin to honestly reflect on those parts of myself that I was so disconnected from. How could I be so knowledgeable academically about addiction, yet still be so out of control with my behaviors? The only possible answer to this was that there was a huge part of my own psyche that was in control of my life that I knew nothing about. At that moment, I finally had my egoic arrogance beaten down enough to admit this.

As I did, so must you. I am not saying you will be as disconnected from yourself as I have been, or that you have been the victim of any type of sexual abuse. What I am saying is that regardless of all that, in order for any of us to have a healthy relationship with sex and sexuality, we must become brutally honest with ourselves. We must become unequivocally intimate with our own personhood as sex and sexuality is the expression of that self-intimacy. It is the surrendering of ego in the presence of another; it is another's surrendering of ego in the presence of you, and there is nothing more intimate than that.

This level of intimacy requires being present with each of our distressing emotions, bearing witness to them, and sharing them with another. Our partners should do the same. Sexual betrayal can be catastrophic for non-addict partners. They struggle with the idea of having sex with someone else without forming an emotional connection to that person. They cannot comprehend the addict's ability to fracture off parts of themselves. To make it even more emotionally distressing, you may not understand how you could have done this either. To understand what we need to do moving forward, we have to relearn how to relate to ourselves and sexuality.

For myself, I had been trained to relate to sex with two references. The first of which was to be wanted, desired, and to bring the other to climax. The second was to be ashamed and hide your true sexual preferences from those who are closest to you. To further muddle the waters, our culture portrays sex as an expression of our innermost committed self, and that it should not be discussed with anyone. I became an object, and I objectified others, which perpetuated a trauma-based relationship with sex. You may not have a trauma-based relationship to sex. It may be based on another distressing emotional process, but make no mistake about it; your relationship to sex and sexuality has been skewed, and you must fundamentally restructure your relationship to it.

Healthy Sex and Sexuality

We are obsessed with sex and sexuality. It is a wonderful expression of ourselves. The act is physically pleasurable, it's how we define our relational status, and yet, it terrifies us. As a society, we have manufactured rigid behavioral requirements around it; we have created boxes for everyone to fit in, and if a person doesn't fit that box, we declare them sexually deviant or perverted. These rigid, harsh ideals and constructs have left a wake of emotional and psychological damage that permeates every culture on every continent.

What I am about to share are a few foundational components of sexual behaviors. To cover all the different aspects of healthy sex and sexuality are beyond the scope of this section. It would take a much longer book to give justice to the plethora of research on the subject.

As a Certified Sex Addiction Therapist (CSAT) and a certified Mindfulness-Based Addiction & Trauma Therapist (MBATT), I acknowledge that there are two camps on the topic of sex and sexuality in the field of psychology: Certified Sex Addiction Therapists and Certified Sex Therapists.

Both camps have much to say about what they see as healthy or harmful sexual behaviors. Each camp claims to know what is "sex positive" or "sex negative," and they debate intensely with one another about this, a debate which is beyond the scope of this section. This field is currently under investigation. Determining what is healthy sexually should be an individual decision. As a result, a therapist should not be prescriptive about what is healthy sex. Rather, a therapist needs to allow the client the opportunity to sit with the distressful emotions they experience around sex in order for the client to mindfully decide what is best for themselves. Further, I would clarify very strongly that no religious ideology should ever inform our perspective on what is healthy sex, and I say that as a working professional in the field. If you have a religious philosophy that informs the way you see sex and sexuality, that is wonderful. I believe the role of a therapist is different as we are, by definition, health care practitioners, and therefore, scientists. When working in our professional capacity, our job is to look at the data and determine what works and what doesn't.

Chapter 7: Sex

Sex is one of two things: a reference to a person's reproductive organs or the act of intercourse. The latter is generally done with another person, but masturbation counts as well. This seems straightforward, so how is it that we have many arguments, banter, and emotions around the idea of sex? We have placed much importance on sex, as we should. Having sex with the person we care about is a wonderfully beautiful act. It can be a dutiful act, with carnal desires being embraced. With sex, we can embrace our conservative or value-driven nature as well. Sex is a behavior that allows us to fully express our attributes with those we love.

The physical act of sex involves multiple domains—ego, awareness, and mind. Here, we can define ego as that which is in relation to everything around us, that which has form, and the projection of what we perceive through our senses. We surrender ego and are at one with all that is around us during these wonderfully intimate moments. There is awareness, the part of ourselves not confined to the restriction of body or language, that part which lies beyond physical expression. Then we have the mind—the internal sense organ—which takes in data and outputs ideas for the ego and awareness.

Our definition of healthy sex must be born out of the integration of these three qualities: mind, ego, and awareness. We must be comfortable with the body and its desire for carnal pleasure. We must fully embrace the projections of the mind, speak, and share them openly with our lover and ourselves. Lastly, we must have an awareness of the emotions that arise for us, and our partners while sharing a sexual experience. Healthy sex is the integration of each of these aspects of ourselves with another.

There are many ways this integration might be expressed. Many sexual fantasies may be played out, or carnal experiences experimented with. Each is beautiful and wonderful as long as it is done and experienced with awareness, leaving no injury, and violating no boundary.

As you can see from the perspective that is being argued here, you may have healthy sex if you are a puritan, a swinger, or if you are attracted to fetishes. It is all fine as long as you are doing so with integrated awareness and honesty. Many will find this alignment difficult, and those who were sexually traumatized will find it especially challenging. However, if one is in awareness and integrated with themselves, their body, and their partner, the specific act(s) of the sexual experience is not as important as the trusting nature of vulnerability that has been embraced while participating in the act(s). One can experience this vulnerable integration only after they have cultivated intimacy and trust with themselves and those around them.

If struggling with sex addiction, I encourage my clients to abstain from orgasm for a period of time—thirty, sixty, or ninety days. Understandably, they become upset, as sex is their most important need. Many of my liberal clients become irate; they believe a hidden, conservative agenda is being imposed upon them. That is not the case. I have found that by taking temporary breaks from sexual activity, many buried emotions, and fractured pieces of one's self come to the surface. The abstinence period provides the space needed to rethink sexual behaviors. For addicts, this is extremely important since the need for sex is all-controlling, dictating when, where, and with whom to have it.

THE FOUR BRAHMA VIHARAS

Healthy sex starts with self-intimacy. To have this, we must cultivate the following:

- Metta: Loving Kindness
- Karuna: Compassion
- Mudita: Sympathetic Joy
- Upekkha: Equanimity

These four qualities are not mindstates, nor are they emotions. They are the natural baseline of the mind when we are not tied to delusional mindsets. *Metta* (loving kindness) and *karuna* (compassion) have been discussed in previous chapters. We will briefly review them here. *Mudita* (sympathetic joy) will be discussed in this section as well, and you will see that it is a different shade of the first two viharas. With consistent practice of the first three viharas, we gain the fourth—*upekkha* (equanimity)—which will be discussed in the last chapter.

Metta—Loving Kindness

Metta is the foundation of intimacy. Only through consistent loving kindness can we truly get to know ourselves. Loving kindness is not a practice of merely accepting our behaviors or indifference. Loving kindness is an open friendliness for our struggles. It's an open understanding that the discomfort we feel by getting to know ourselves is a sign of our progression on the path of recovery. This friendliness is something that must be practiced. Just as a new runner cannot finish a marathon, an addict new to recovery cannot provide loving kindness from the get-go. The runner and the addict must practice for a period of time to reach that point. For the addict, the practice can be as simple as greeting those you see throughout the day and offering a smile to anyone you encounter. One could even offer a smile to themselves each time they look in a mirror. Every time you notice a rigid or judgmental thought, you can take one breath and respond to the rigidness with friendliness. If we notice a harsh attitude or an aversive mindset to something or someone, we take contrary thoughts and embrace them with friendliness.

Addicts need loving kindness for the idea that they are addicts. We need to embrace all parts of ourselves with friendliness. Friendliness doesn't mean we grant permission for the addict's mind to run amok. It means we don't hold onto aversive mindstates; we don't shy away from the discomfort that arises from our awareness that we are, in fact, addicts. We continue to smile and help ourselves, just as we would help a close friend.

Karuna—Compassion

Compassion is cultivated through the focus of the mind and can be categorized into two types—destructive and constructive.

Destructive compassion is exemplified by the following: Let's say you come across an active alcoholic who asks you for money outside of a liquor store. We may feel deep sadness and pain due to their struggle, and we might offer them money, which we know will help them buy a drink. After all, if they don't have the object of their desire, they will suffer. This is destructive compassion and is based on ignorance. If we were to utilize the wise mind, we would understand that in the long run, this only promotes their addiction and suffering.

Alternatively, we could choose to have constructive compassion by letting the alcoholic know that we cannot offer them money, but we can offer them a ride to a recovery center that will address the cause of their suffering. The addict will likely decline, which may leave you saddened, pained, or relieved, all of which are fine reactions. Remember, emotions are natural and normal, and they are to be embraced with loving kindness.

How do we focus the mind in order to cultivate compassion? Many exercises exist, and focused meditation is an efficient way to start. We begin by focusing the mind on someone we truly love. We repeat the words in our mind:

May they have love,

may they have compassion,

may they be free of suffering.

We repeat this many times over, at every chance we get. In the meditation chapter, you learned that meditation is completed lying down, sitting, standing up, or moving. If we come across a person who is upset with us, we can repeat the mantra of compassion in our heads. When we have someone in front of us in line that's taking forever, we can repeat the mantra to ourselves. This is what makes compassion a verb.

We can build on our training by focusing our minds on a friend or loved one. Hold them in your mind and repeat the compassion mantra:

CHAPTER 7: SEX

May they have love,

may they have compassion,

may they be free of suffering.

As we progress in our ability to do this, we can train further by picking random people who are neutral to us. Maybe we do not even know them—it could be someone just walking down the street. If we are feeling like living on the edge, we may hold that person in our minds all day long and offer them compassion. When we see them, we begin to think the thoughts:

May they have compassion,

may they have love,

may they be free from suffering.

We can focus this mantra on ourselves as well:

May I have compassion,

may I have love,

may I be free from suffering,

As our practice progresses, we come to a point where we think of people we do not like. We may have a family member who was mean to us or perhaps a co-worker who rubs us the wrong way. Whoever it is, we hold that person in our mind's eye and repeat:

May they have compassion,

may they have love,

may they be free from suffering.

We do this repeatedly, and this practice can last a lifetime. It does not repress feelings of anger or pain that we may have experienced in relation to this person. Instead, we allow ourselves to feel those powerful, edgy feelings, and yet, we still offer loving compassion to that person! Use the person's name whenever possible. When an addict is triggered, they can repeat the mantra of compassion to themselves in response to their aggressive focus.

With all of this in mind, let's ask again—what is healthy sex? Beyond the integration of mind, awareness, and ego that we discussed, the question demands further exploration. Religious fundamentalism deems certain aspects of sex as sacred, while other aspects may be considered immoral. A sexually liberal person may see things differently. When the dust settles, the only clear thing is that healthy sex is subjective. As addicts, we must keep the following in mind:

- All human interaction involves emotion. To have healthy sex, we must be present with the emotions that arise from sexual interactions.

- Healthy sex involves physical interaction. It involves sharing your body. This includes masturbation, which is sharing your body with yourself.

- Healthy sex is honest; there are no lies in the action or intention of either party.

- Healthy sex is not physically harmful; you are not causing serious physical harm to another.

People may disagree about the last point, and that is okay. If you enjoy sexual acts with themes of sadism or masochism, that is fine as long as it is done safely. But if a person states they want to be tied to a rack and electrocuted with a car battery charger or somehow tortured in a manner that risks true harm, such as having a plastic bag placed over their head in a process called autoerotic asphyxiation, I would say that this is NOT healthy. These acts place both the giver and receiver at great risk. The person receiving may be injured for life or die (which has occurred many times), and the person providing the torture risks a lifetime of guilt and incarceration.

At this point, people will say to me, "If that's what they want to do, isn't that up to them?" I will answer by telling them that our culture has decided that it's not up to them.

For example, if a person wants to jump off a bridge to die, we do not accept this, and we strive to prevent this type of behavior from happening. Sexual behaviors that are self-injurious are no different. This is not my opinion; this is what we, in the West, as a culture, have collectively come to decide. I am not arguing right or wrong, good or bad. I am simply stating what is.

To summarize our journey through this topic, healthy sex incorporates aconnection to emotion, honesty, and causes no harm. It does not violate our personal values. It is about vulnerability, connection, and a lustful, joyous, pleasurable surrender to our desires and the desires of others. It explores our bodies, our partner's body (or bodies), and does so in a safe manner—participants are able to make clear and mindful choices for themselves about whether they want to continue to participate in sex or not. This does not mean sex cannot be passionate, dark, or even carnal; it very much can be. We can take part in these pleasures within the limits and boundaries we and society have set for us.

The idea of behaving sexually within the limits and boundaries set by society is tricky; as a gay man, I know how thorny this can be. Many societies still punish homosexuality with death, and there are still pockets of the United States that find it acceptable to beat and punish those who are gay or send them to camps to be cured. When I talk about the boundaries society has set for us, I am referring to the idea of doing no harm. This may be a value that we need to take ownership of, and not so much one imposed by society.

Lastly, I will say that the ultimate decider of what is healthy for you is you! How do you want your sex life to be? What do you want from your sexual relations? These choices can only be made after a long process of gaining self-introspection, awareness, and compassion. You must figure this out with a therapist. I would again encourage you to see a Certified Mindfulness-Based Addiction & Trauma Therapist or a Certified Sex Addiction Therapist. I would even recommend a Certified Sex Therapist. If you are seeing a Certified Sex Therapist, I encourage you to be sure that they understand sexual addiction. If you are seeing a Certified Sex Addiction Therapist, I recommend that they are someone who is sex positive and does not allow their own religious ideology or personal values to be prescriptive about how you relate to sex.

MUDITA: SYMPATHETIC JOY

If you pour a handful of salt into a cup of water, the water becomes undrinkable. But if you pour the salt into a river, people can continue to draw the water to cook, wash, and drink. The river is immense and it has the capacity to receive, embrace, and transform. When our hearts are small, our understanding and

compassion are limited, and we suffer. We cannot accept or tolerate others and their shortcomings, and we demand that they change. But when our hearts expand and the same things don't make us suffer anymore, we have a lot of understanding and compassion and can embrace others, we accept others as they are, and they have the chance to transform. So, the question is, how do we allow our hearts to grow?
—Thich Nhat Hanh

As we progress with our recovery, we gain awareness of the changes we have made. Our continued practice of recovery moves us away from the rigid self-destructive mindset we had and allows us to increase a gentle awareness of the pain we've caused others and ourselves.

Buddhist monk, Thich Nhat Hanh, is expressing the idea that if you are suffering, you have fallen victim to the tyranny of the fixated mind. As we feel pain, be it physical or emotional, the mind tightens and disconnects from the world around it and fixates on that pain. The result of this tightening is the mind generates hypotheses that become increasingly delusional. The mind claims that we are "going to feel this forever." It will spit out ideas related to absolutes and try to convince us that we are somehow broken.

I want to restate here that none of us are terminally unique. We can heal if we want to, but we must be mindful of the need to actively reconnect ourselves to reality. We must uncouple this "fixated mind" and reconnect to the reality of the current moment. We must begin to increase the container that we see ourselves in. This is where the idea of "letting go and letting your higher power take control" in 12-step programs comes from. It does not matter to me what vernacular we use; we can call this process "letting go and letting god;" we can remind ourselves we are part of the universe, or we can take on a hardcore scientific relationship to this idea of being the universe. After all, the universe and our bodies are made of the same thing—space! This view allows us to see that we are not fixed to this moment in time. We can also increase the container we are in by connecting to others and asking for their loving support.

When I say others, I am referring to people who are in recovery and who are sober; people who have or are actively learning to love themselves in a healthy way. It is only by increasing our perception of interconnectedness that we are ever able to make it through those tyrannical moments of the addictive mind.

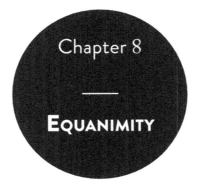

Chapter 8

EQUANIMITY

We had been shopping all day, spending what I felt was a ton of money. My mom and I walked into a large warehouse store, the lights shining brightly on different pieces of furniture that I could not afford. At this time, my mom was retired, and she had done quite well for herself, but for her to spend this much was troublesome for me. I remember how each thing she purchased moved me closer to the shame and guilt I felt inside for being unable to care for myself at the age of forty.

Here I was, a grown man starting over completely due to addiction, and my mom was coming to my rescue the best way she knew how. Yet, the more she spent on me, the greater the densely dark ball of shame in the pit of my stomach became. Recalling this now, I still feel its heaviness; even today, I am working to embrace my worthiness.

We walked through the enormous store, and my mom was in her element—she loves to (in her words), "Buy, not shop." We were looking at mattresses, and she asked which one I wanted. I told her I was having a hard time accepting this gift from her; she had already done so much for me. She assured me not to worry and asked again which mattress I wanted. She told me to lie down on several kinds and tell her which one I liked. I asked the salesperson for the cheapest mattress they had and insisted on getting it.

She then asked me, "Is that the one you feel most comfortable on?" Now I was in real trouble, as I could not lie to her. Sitting on the cheapest mattress in the store, I looked at her in silence, flooded with shame. She asked me what was wrong.

I responded, "Mom, this is too much."

She smiled and said, "You know, your father has the same reaction when I go out to buy things, so I will tell you what I tell him." She pointed to another part of the store and said, "Go over there while I take care of this. I can tell you like the other one, so just go on, and I will find you later."

I did as instructed.

I learned much about the power of shame that afternoon. I could not see it before, but I could see it then. What my mom was doing for me is what any mom would do for their child: she was helping me build a foundation on which I could take care of myself. She was offering me the gift she offered me when I was a child. She was not taking responsibility for me as an adult. She was simply saying that I was her son, and she loved me.

The deep shame I carried from making destructive choices was interfering with my ability to be present and thankful to my mother at that moment. It took me approximately six months in therapy to realize this.

Even though several years have passed, I still feel that wonderful wash of shame just thinking about it. Accepting these gifts from my mother on that day forced me to confront my shame. Over time, I realized that the feeling has nothing to do with my lovability; it is just a natural part of being human. Does my mind still have thoughts that arise out of that emotional energy? Of course. However, now I am able to see that those thoughts are just based on the childhood abuse I experienced, and are in no way related to my value as a human being.

To be non-reactively present with our emotions requires an understanding of the last of the Four Brahma-vihara: equanimity.

Aligning with Realitiy

The process of recovery is not about changing who we are; it is not about moving away from any thoughts or emotional states; and it is not about finding a way to deny, replace, or even extinguish the emotional distress we feel as we go about our daily lives. The process of recovery is about opening up to any and all emotional states, allowing ourselves to align with the reality that everything in the universe is exactly as it should be at this time.

The mind is highly aversive to this process and always wants to create thoughts that are wrapped in delusion. Yes, all mindstates are delusion, but when we can let go of acting on those mindstates, we can learn to live and align with whatever arises. There is no point in not aligning with open arms to each moment, no matter how pleasurable or distressing it may be.

At this point, you may be freaking out, as many of my clients do when they hear this. They say to themselves, "If I move close to those states, I'll be back in active addiction." This is a red herring as I am not telling you to act on the mindstates; I am saying that you must allow yourself to see them, but that you do not need to do anything with them. You must accept that at times there will be urges to engage in certain behaviors, and at other times, there won't. Whenever we experience either possibility, we simply allow ourselves to see them, witness them, and know that they will pass.

This "knowing they will pass" is based on the reality that everything in the universe is in a state of perpetual transformation. The moment we are born, we begin to die. The car you drive, the computer you use, and the house you live in are all in a state of decay or change. Even the love you have (or don't have) is constantly evolving. The body you are temporarily in possession of is also not a static object. It may seem as if it is, but in actuality, the body is a process consisting of trillions of events happening simultaneously to maintain the illusions of the body.

The psychiatrist M. Scott Peck once said, "Mental health is the absolute commitment to reality, no matter what the cost." We must come to terms with the impermanence of all things, everything we love or hate, including the urges to act on our addictive impulses, which can be excruciatingly difficult to bear, and at times, we must reach out for help.

If nothing in the universe stays the same, is there anything constant? The answer is yes—change is constant, and therefore, uncertainty is constant.

Often times, clients I see come to a point in their treatment where they express confusion, and it is at this moment that I become flooded with joy because that's what the process is all about. Confusion is a glimpse into the plane of infinite possibility, and that is the only thing real in the universe. The idea that everything is in flux means that potentiality is all that there really is—the prospect of a new event, or not knowing what is next. That confusion is a wonderful sign that we only have now, and the only thing that we know for certain is this moment.

Every sun, planet, gravitational wave, black hole, every bit of dark matter, and dark energy—everything known and unknown had to happen exactly as it has for this moment to be as it is; this moment will never happen the same way again, and once it passes, everything is different. This moment—here and now—is a miracle, no matter how distressing our mind wants it to be.

I am not denying anyone's pain. We don't need to instantly feel good about times when we were violated. As someone who experienced rape twice and was molested repeatedly as a child, I would never minimize the pain of such events. They are immensely painful and need not ever be minimized, but our only wise choice is to move into that pain and allow ourselves to feel it.

This is not done easily, and it can never be done alone. We must always reach out to others, and we must always share the pain and allow ourselves to be loved in a healthy manner. We must realize that the pain, sadness, joy, anger, shame, fear, or guilt of any event will come and go. If we are in equanimity, we are able to simply be aware of this. We simply see the emotional energy rise, crest, and fall like a wave in the ocean. We need not be reactionary in an effort to make it go away (aversion) or hold onto it (clinging). Reactionary behavior will do the opposite of what we want:

uncomfortable emotions will persist while wanted emotions will dissipate quickly.

Calm in the Eye of a Hurricane

Imagine you were in a car accident, resulting in a pole going through your neck where it is now stuck. You are rushed to the ER and have a choice of two doctors: both are equally qualified, though neither has treated a patient with a pole running through their neck.

Doctor A comes in and exclaims, "Oh my God! You have a pole in your neck! Nurse, come quick, call someone, we have to do something!"

Doctor B comes in calmly, appearing methodical and collected. He says, "We are going to take care of you. I know you may be scared, but don't worry. My team and I will take care of this."

You would undoubtedly choose the calm doctor whose calmness would be essential to your survival. The upset and rattled doctor would naturally increase your fear, heart rate, and blood pressure—all factors that are not helpful in this scenario.

Part of what allows me to be a good therapist is my ability to be the calm, collected voice in the room. It does not mean that I am not feeling the fear, anger, shame, and guilt in the room; quite the opposite, I am feeling each emotion deeply.

However, I have cultivated the ability to have equanimity in the room when those emotions are pervasive.

This is what we must all eventually learn to do, and it doesn't happen overnight, nor will it be easy. Living in addiction, however, is also not easy. Think of the cost, cover-ups, and sickness compounded on one another, leaving us isolated, broke, lost, in poor health, utterly disconnected from reality.

Total and complete acceptance of each moment—with loving compassion and a deep connection to our experience—allows a freedom that is simply not possible to have in any other way. Equanimity is a quality that naturally arises out of this open connection to what is—regardless of how distressing or pleasurable it may be. We do not need to do anything to gain it; equanimity naturally arises out of our continued practice of mindfulness and compassion.

Equanimity is a combination of power, presence, and strength. These are the three legs of the stool that we need to have a balanced life. As we journey on, we will have contrasting experiences, which in Buddhism are known as the *eight worldly winds*:

- Fame and Disrepute
- Gain and Loss
- Pleasure and Pain
- Praise and Blame

Whatever or however we want to say it, shit happens in life, and there is nothing we can do about it. Some of it we like and some we don't. Equanimity is about allowing ourselves to have a deep relationship with all of these things—shitty or not—by leaning into it without reactivity. Practicing allows us the grand ability to be present with ourselves and our emotions, and we gain a greater ability to be closer to others when they have their own experiences.

When we are calm and compassionate, a domino effect occurs: we are able to be closer to ourselves, closer to others, better able to love and allow ourselves to be loved. Some call this a reciprocally deterministic relationship. As we wake up to this quality of balance, a natural wisdom begins to permeate from us.

No one likes loss or blame while everyone enjoys pleasure and gain, but since the reality is that nothing stays forever, don't delude yourself. In those moments of pleasure, take a deep breath and acknowledge it. When pain arises, take a deep breath and acknowledge it as well. This is all we must do.

Equanimty does not equate to indifference, which is a sense of denial—a pretending that we *don't care*. With equanimity, we can simply be with our emotions honestly, openly, and with compassion and wisdom. This takes a lifetime, and if you believe in the Buddhist idea of reincarnation, it may take hundreds of lifetimes. This is okay; those seasons of our life are going to happen regardless, so it is best to accept them with gentle, loving compassion. Resisting only leads to more suffering, and we know this without a doubt because we have been resisting reality for most of our lives, allowing addiction to run amok. We must now learn to sit in the middle of all the turmoil, and through this action, we begin to see the true power of our practice.

Not until I was forty years old, did I realize that one's home should be a place of peace and gentleness. I was still an intern at the time of this epiphany, and after a long day's work, I would come home to my small studio apartment across from the beach. It was my first home after I got out of the hospital from my drug overdose. My mom had come down when I moved in, bringing me kitchenware and taking me shopping for furniture, as I mentioned earlier.

After a particularly difficult day at work, I came home and was greeted by my chihuahua, Pema. I sat down on the futon, took a deep breath, and felt all the tension leave my body as an ocean breeze came through the window. At that moment, I had such gratitude to be home, and the awakening of this gratitude stunned me. For the first time, I understood what people meant when they said, "Your home should be a sanctuary." I called my mom and told her of this realization that was forty years in the making.

She giggled and lovingly said, "Well, of course it has to be. Otherwise, a person would go crazy!"

I am still amazed that it took forty years for a basic concept to come to my awareness. I am also filled with joy that it did. Having a sanctuary is part of the bedrock you must create to build a loving relationship with yourself. If you have family and children, you need to set a good example for them by caring for yourself. Create a place at home that is a sanctuary for you to relax in and meditate each day.

Being gentle with yourself is not ingesting substances that intoxicate and harm you. For instance, alcohol is a poison that is filtered out by the liver, and if the liver cannot excrete that poison fast enough, it builds up in the blood, makes its way to the brain, and you become intoxicated. Pills work much the same way. Abstaining from intoxicating substances is not about judgment; it is about treating yourself and your body in a loving manner.

Being gentle with yourself is the achievement of balance. It's taking into account acceptance, mind, the practice of meditation, compassion, awareness, honesty, intimacy, and equanimity of it all. Being gentle with yourself is awakening from the addictive mind and choosing a life in recovery. Being gentle with yourself is the behavioral expression of your acceptance of the lovability that you know you have. Now, think about that last sentence carefully—nowhere did it say that your mind has to agree. In fact, the mind has nothing to do with it. You must go and behave as if the mind already knows you are lovable. Thus, you must *behave gently with yourself*.

REFERENCES

Chapter 1:

Bien, T. *Mindful Therapy: A Guide for Therapists and Helping Professionals*. Wisdom Publications. 2006.

Burnett, H. *BBC Face To Face*. Interview with Carl Jung. 1959.

Carnes, P. *Facing the Shadow*, 1st edition. Gentle Path Press. 2001.

Carnes, P. *Out of the Shadows*, 3rd edition. Hazelden. 2001.

Eagleman, D. *Incognito: The Secret Lives of the Brain*. Pantheon. 2011.

Eurich, T. *Insight: Why we are not as self-aware as we think and how seeing ourselves clearly helps us succeed at work and in life* (Audiobook). Random House. 2017.

Ford, J. B. *Auto Process Therapy Treatment Model and Practice: An Original Buddhist Psychotherapy*. Authorhouse. 2014.

Segal, Z.V., Williams, J.G., & Teasdale, J.D. *Mindfulness-Based Cognitive Therapy for Depression: A New Approach to Preventing Relapse*. The Guilford press. 2002.

Sucitto, A. *Meditation—A Way of Awakening*. Amaravati Publications. 2011.

Weiss, R. *Why Buddhism is True*. Simon & Schuster. 2017.

Chapter 2:

Somerville, L.H. *Searching for signatures of brain maturity: what are we searching for?* Neuron. Volume 92, Issue 6, December 2016.

Jerath, R. & Crawford, M.W. *Layers of human brain activity: a functional model based on the default mode network and slow oscillations*. Frontiers of Human Neuroscience. April 2015.

Koob, G.F. & Volkow, N.D. *Neurobiology of addiction: a neurocircuitry analysis*. The Lancet Psychiatry. Volume 3, Issue 8, August 2016.

Chapter 3:
Knapen, J., Vancampfort, D., Moriën, Y., & Marchal, Y. *Exercise therapy improves both mental and physical health in*

patients with major depression. Disability and Rehabilitation. Volume 37, 2015—Issue 16.

Davis, R. *Craving, desire and addiction*. Presentation at XXVII Mind and Life Institute Conference.

Chapter 5:

Fogel, A. *Emotional and physical pain activate similar brain regions*. Psychology Today. Apr 19, 2012.

Thaler, R. & Sunstein, C.R. *Nudge: Improving Decisions about Health, Wealth, and Happiness*. Yale University Press. 2008.
Chapter 6:

Seligman, M. E. P. *Learned helplessness*. Annual Review of Medicine. 23 (1): 407–412. 1972.

Chapter 8:

Peck, M.S. *The Road Less Traveled*, 25th Anniversary Edition: A New Psychology of Love, Traditional Values, and Spiritual Growth. Deckle Edge. 2002.

Note from the Author:

After the completion of this book, I received feedback from family members. I would like to clarify a few things: the human mind and the memories we form in our younger years can often confuse and conflate different events into a narrative that may not be identical to those who were also present for the same event.

For example, after speaking with my sister (who is four years older than me), I learned that my father beat my mother with the phone receiver in the kitchen, not the living room. This was surprising as my memory of this event was different, as depicted in this book.

My stepmom, Laura, and brother, Jeff, also informed me that the fight in the garage started because Laura witnessed my father throwing a socket wrench at my brother's head. According to my stepmom, my dad did not punch her, but he did slap her.

I felt compelled to put this note into the book to be as transparent and honest as possible. What I expressed are my memories. They may not be 100 percent accurate; however, the traumatic effect on my development is 100 percent accurate. My hope is that this allows survivors of childhood trauma to understand that just because the experience you had may be confused and/or different than what those around you experienced, it does not necessarily mean that you are mistaken. This is how the human mind forms memories when we are children. It folds events into a narrative, and that narrative may not be exact. The overall theme of the event, however, will match the theme of those who also experienced that event.

Acknowledgments:

I am deeply grateful for those who have helped me with the completion of this book.

I acknowledge and thank Chris Bordey for his design and layout work on this project. He has helped me more than words can say.

I thank Christian Quebral for his notational editing, research, and project management. More importantly, I thank Christian for challenging me to dig deeper and be more vulnerable in my writing.

I thank Jordana Berliner for her encouragement and the refinement she brought to this project. I am grateful for her support.

Last, but not least, I want to thank my niece Britney Humphries, who not only held me to task but coordinated the chaos of my mind into the symmetry needed to communicate pithy ideas.

ALSO BY DARRIN FORD:

Transforming the Addictive Mind, 2017
& *Recovery Coaching Client Handbook*, 2018

AVAILABLE AT SANOPRESS.COM

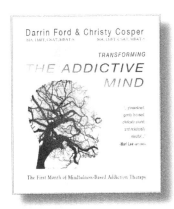 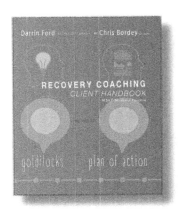

The Mindful Addict, video blog, 2020

THE MINDFUL ADDICT (DARRIN FORD) DISCUSSES CURRENT EVENTS AND HOW IT RELATES TO ADDICTION AND RECOVERY.

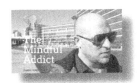 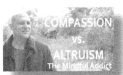 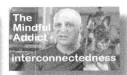

ABOUT THE AUTHOR

Darrin Ford, LMFT, CSAT-S, MBATT-S is certified by the American Association of Marriage and Family Therapists as a Clinical Supervisor of Associate Therapists. As founder of *Mindful Centers for Addiction and Trauma Therapy*, he has integrated mindfulness into the treatment of those struggling with addiction. He has also worked mentoring therapists in the utilization of mindfulness and the development of their private practice. In addition, Darrin is a nationally recognized speaker and internationally published author. His books include *Transforming the Addictive Mind* and *The Recovery Coaching Client Handbook*.

In his spare time, Darrin enjoys watching sci-fi movies and action shows. He often travels back to his hometown in Needles, California to visit family. He enjoys spending time with his partner, Chris, and their chihuahua, Amos. Together, they live in Long Beach, California.

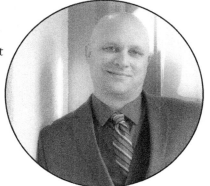

You may contact Darrin at: www.darrinford.com

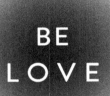

Made in the USA
Coppell, TX
01 October 2020

39141123R00105